GW00402095

OVER-THE-COUNTER DRUGS

OVER-THE-COUNTER DRUGS

Dr D G Delvin

MB BS LRCP MRCS DOBST
RCOG DCH FPA CERT
MRCGP DIP VEN
MFFP

The ROYAL
SOCIETY of
MEDICINE

SUNBURST BOOKS

Editorial Advisor

DR KATHARINE A ORTON
MB BS MRCGP
DCH DRCOG

Author's Acknowledgement
I would like to express my sincere thanks to my
pharmaceutical advisor, Jo Grimes, M.R.Pharm.S.

This edition first published in 1995 by
Sunburst Books, Deacon House,
65 Old Church Street, London SW3 5BS.

Copyright
Text © David Delvin 1995
Layout and design © Sunburst Books 1995

ISBN 1 85778 163 5

Printed and bound in China

CONTENTS

INTRODUCTION

Welcome to our guide to 'over-the-counter' medications – in other words, things you can buy at the chemist **without** a doctor's prescription.

In most countries, very powerful drugs, and especially those which have a lot of potentially serious side-effects, are kept 'on prescription'.

But in recent years, there has been a general tendency to ease the restrictions and make more products available over-the-counter. For example, the strong anti-acid drugs Tagamet, Zantac and Pepcid have lately become available over-the-counter in some countries – though with certain limitations on the way they are used.

This trend can go too far: for instance, there are many parts of the world where it is legal to buy powerful antibiotics which can have disastrous ill-effects if they are misused. But in general, it is a good thing that the public can now buy a wide range of medications to treat minor illnesses, without having to see a doctor first.

However, do please read the health warnings on the following page, because it is important to understand that buying over-the-counter drugs is not entirely free of risk.

What is the best way to use this book? I suggest that if you have a health problem (such as acne, a cold, indigestion, or whatever), you begin by looking it up in the contents, and then turn to the appropriate section.

Each section begins with some brief introductory advice; please read it – particularly as it will alert you to any special problems with the types of medication described in that section.

Next, you will find a list of OTC preparations which can be used for that particular problem. In many cases, I have listed the ingredients contained in the product. This information is worth knowing for three reasons:

* A lot of products with different brand names contain exactly the same ingredients. You may well decide to choose the cheapest one.

* When you look at the ingredients of a product, you may recognise one that has done you good in the past.

* In contrast, you may recognise the name of an ingredient that has done you harm in the past; for instance, you may be allergic to it. In these circumstances you should choose a different product which does not contain the ingredient.

I do hope you find this little book useful. Before you dip into it, please make sure you read and understand the warning notes below.

Dr David Delvin

HEALTH WARNINGS

* All drugs can have side-effects – and that applies to every medication in this book.

* Many drugs can 'interact' with other drugs. So if you are already on any medication, DO NOT buy an over-the-counter product unless the pharmacist tells you that it is safe to use the two things at the same time.

* If anything unusual occurs when you are using a product, STOP using it at once and contact your doctor or pharmacist for advice.

* If you are pregnant, or trying to get pregnant, DO NOT use any medication unless your doctor assures you that it is safe to do so.

* If you are breast-feeding a baby, do not take any medication which hasn't been approved by your doctor.

* When buying any OTC medication, always ask the pharmacist's advice about how to use it.

* Always read the label – and any instructions that come with the product.

* Never exceed the stated dose. Taking more is unlikely to do you more good – and may do you serious harm.

* When reading this book, please bear in mind that manufacturers sometimes change the names – and the contents – of their products. So be guided by the advice you are given by the pharmacist at the time.

* The content of a product sometimes varies from country to country. So always check the label – and be guided by the pharmacist.

ACNE AND SPOTS

General Advice

Acne and spots are very common. In fact, most teenage boys and girls experience some degree of acne at times.

There is no clear distinction between having acne and having spots. Many doctors regard having a few spots as being *mild* acne. If you only have a few spots which do not trouble you much, then it is reasonable to buy a remedy from the chemist's.

However, most dermatologists (doctors who specialise in skin disorders) do not set great store by over-the-counter preparations for acne. Instead they would suggest that if you have moderate or severe acne, you should begin by going to your general practitioner.

She will probably put you on a long course of an antibiotic (courses of only a few weeks are often useless), perhaps prescribing tetracycline or erythromycin, and a powerful skin application such as Retin-A.

In very severe cases your GP may send you to a hospital dermatologist, who could prescribe the strong anti-acne drug Roaccutane. However, this can have major side-effects.

In contrast, over-the-counter preparations (listed below) are generally very mild. However, those that contain benzoyl peroxide can cause some stinging, and possibly dryness and peeling of your skin.

Most of the over-the-counter remedies are intended either to reduce the number of germs on your skin, or to clear out 'plugs' from your pores.

Please do not expect any overnight miracles from the products listed below. It is usually necessary to use these preparations long-term to achieve any real effect.

Over-the-counter preparations for acne include:

Acetoxyl 2.5, and 5 Gels containing benzoyl peroxide. Acetoxyl 5 is twice as strong as Acetoxyl 2.5. Apply once daily after washing with soap and water.

Acne Aid Soap A special soap with no colourants or perfumes that might irritate the skin. Use to make a lather, then wash. Avoid the eyes.

Acnegel and Acnegel Forte These are gels containing 5% and 10% benzoyl peroxide respectively. Apply once daily after washing.

Acnidazil A non-greasy 'vanishing cream' containing benzoyl peroxide and an anti-fungal agent. Follow directions on label. Try on a small area first.

Benoxyl 5, and 10 Lotions containing benzoyl peroxide in 5% and 10% strengths respectively. Apply once daily after washing.

Benzagel 5, and 10 Gels containing 5% and 10% benzoyl peroxide respectively. Apply once daily after washing.

Betadine Scalp and Skin Cleanser Contains a form of iodine intended to kill germs. Follow directions on bottle. Do not use if sensitive to iodine.

Biactol Liquid Germ-killing facewash. Use instead of soap, morning and night.

Blake's Veil Cover Cream Excellent 'camouflage' product, very useful for temporarily disguising a bad acne spot. Available in a wide range of tints, to match any skin shade.

Brasivol Cleansing and abrading agent, available in two strengths: 'Fine 1' and 'Medium 2'. Rub on three or four times daily.

Cepton Gel Contains an antiseptic. Rub on a thin layer, morning and evening.

Cepton Lotion Blue lotion, containing the same antiseptic as Cepton Gel *(see above)*.

Cepton Medicated Skin Wash Red fluid, containing the same antiseptic as Cepton Gel *(see above)*.

Clearasil Cream containing sulphur and triclosan.

Apply twice daily after washing. Available in colour-less or tinted forms.

Clearasil Dual Action Pads Cleansing pads containing 2% salicylic acid.

Clearasil Medicated Cover Stick Cosmetic stick, useful for camouflaging blackheads and spots.

Clearasil Medicated Face Wash Liquid containing 0.7% phenoxypropanol.

Clearasil Medicated Lotion Contains alcohol, a detergent and two antiseptics.

Clearasil Medicated Milk Contains alcohol, a surfactant and ergosan.

Clearasil Soap Coconut soap bar, containing ergosan.

Clearasil Medicated Moisturiser Moisturiser containing triclosan.

Eskamel Cream containing resorcinol and sulphur. Apply sparingly once a day after washing.

Harrogate Sulphur Soap A sulphur-containing soap bar.

Mediclear 10 Cream A cream containing 10% benzoyl peroxide. Apply once daily after washing.

Mediclear Lotion A white lotion containing 5% benzoyl peroxide. Apply once daily after washing.

Oxy 5, and 10 Lotions containing benzoyl peroxide at 5% and 10% strengths respectively. See pack for instructions.

Oxy Clean Facial Scrub A gel containing sodium borate and triclosan. See pack for instructions.

Panoxyl 5, and 10 Gels containing 5% and 10% benzoyl peroxide respectively. Apply once daily after washing.

Panoxyl Aqua Gel A gel containing 2.5% benzoyl peroxide. Apply daily after washing.

Quinoderm Antibacterial Face Wash Blue face wash containing two common antiseptics (cetrimide and chlorhexidine) plus sodium lauroyl sacosinate and lauric diethanolamide. Keep away from eyes.

Quinoderm Cream Cream containing 10% benzoyl peroxide, plus potassium hydroxyquinoline sulphate. Apply sparingly two or three times daily.

Quinoderm Cream 5 Similar to Quindoderm Cream *(see* above*)*, but containing half the strength of benzoyl peroxide.

Quinoderm Lotio-gel 5 per cent Contains the same ingredients as Quindoderm Cream 5 *(see* above*)*. Apply one to three times daily.

Torbetol Blue face lotion containing the antiseptics cetrimide and chlorhexidine. Apply with cotton wool, one to three times daily.

Ultra Clearasil Cream containing benzoyl peroxide. Available in two strengths: 'Maximum' (10%) and 'Regular' (5%), colourless or tinted.

Ultra Clearasil Zit Zapper Applicator containing 10% benzoyl peroxide.

Valderma Cream Cream containing chlorocresol plus potassium hydroxyquinoline sulphate. Apply two or three daily after washing.

Valderma Soap Blue soap containing trichlorocarbonilide. Use in place of normal soap, two or three times a day.

ATHLETE'S FOOT

GENERAL ADVICE

Athlete's foot is an exceedingly common skin infection, particularly among younger men and women. It is caused by a fungus, and for some reason it nearly always attacks the area between the fourth and little toes, though it may spread elsewhere on the foot, and even up the leg.

It does not only affect athletes, though it does tend to be spread around in sports changing rooms and showers. However, it can equally well lurk on your bedroom or kitchen floor.

It causes an itchy flaking of the skin – often referred to by young men as 'foot rot'. If it spreads up the leg, it usually causes little yellow blisters. Sometimes there may be 'rings' of inflammation which extend over the upper surface of the foot.

If athlete's foot is **only** causing trouble between your fourth and fifth toes, then there is little point in going to your doctor about it. Just buy one of the proprietary preparations listed below (you may have to continue with it for some time), and use the following common-sense hygiene measures:

* Don't walk around barefoot – especially in changing rooms and communal showers (if necessary, you can buy shower slippers)

* Always dry between your toes very carefully after bathing or showering

* Don't share towels with anyone else

* Wear a clean pair of socks or tights every day

However, if the infection is clearly spreading on to the top of your foot or on to the sole – or up your

13

legs – then you need to get advice and treatment from a doctor.

Over-the-counter preparations for athlete's foot include:

Anaflex Cream A white foot cream, containing 10% polynoxylin. Apply twice daily.

Canesten Cream Cream (containing 1% clotrimazole), better known for treating thrush infections of the vulva, but also useful against athlete's foot.

Castellani's Paint Old-fashioned remedy, worth a try in long-standing 'dry' athlete's foot which has failed to clear up with other treatments.

Daktarin Cream Powerful cream containing the anti-fungal agent miconazole nitrate (2%). Apply twice daily until about two weeks after all signs of athlete's foot have gone. Discontinue use if you get a sensitivity reaction.

Daktarin Powder Contains the same ingredient as Daktarin Cream *(see* above*)*. Shake between the toes and inside the shoes and socks till two weeks after all signs of infection have gone.

Daktarin Spray Powder Similar in use and effect to Daktarin Powder *(see* above*)*. Do not use on broken skin.

Ecostatin Cream White cream containing the anti-fungal drug econazole nitrate. More useful than powder for 'weeping' patches. Discontinue use if you get any sensitivity reaction.

Ecostatin Lotion Similar to Ecostatin Cream *(see* above*)*, but in the form of a white lotion.

Ecostatin Powder and Spray Powder Both products contain the same ingredient as Ecostatin Cream *(see* previous entry*)*. Do not spray them near the eyes or face.

Ecostatin Spray Solution Contains same ingredient as Ecostatin Cream *(see* above*)*. Keep away from eyes and mouth. Do not inhale.

Germolene Medicated Foot Spray An aerosol containing dichlorophen and triclosan. Spray over the affected area, but not more than five times per day.

Healthy Feet A cream intended to deal with athlete's foot and also 'hot and tired' feet. Contains undeclinic acid and dibromopropamide.

Monphytol Paint Pink liquid containing six ingredients, including methyl salicylate and chlorbutol. Apply twice daily.

Mycil Athlete's Foot Spray Contains the old-established anti-fungal drug, tolnaftate. Use night and morning.

Mycil Ointment Very well known athlete's foot remedy, containing tolnaftate, plus benzalkonium chloride (some people are sensitive to the latter). Apply twice daily.

Mycil Powder Like Mycil Ointment *(see* above*)*. Contains tolnaftate, but no benzalkonium chloride. Also contains the antiseptic chlorhexidine. Apply twice daily.

Mycota A cream containing two related anti-fungal agents: zinc undecenoate and undecenoic acid. Apply twice daily after washing and drying the affected area thoroughly.

Mycota Powder Same ingredients and method of use as Mycota *(see* above*)*, but in slightly different proportions and in powder form.

Mycota Spray Use as for other brands of Mycota. Contains dichlorophen and undecenoic acid.

Permanganate Solution Old-fashioned, non-proprietary remedy for 'weeping' athlete's foot. Your pharmacist will have to make it up specially for you, and instruct you on how to bathe your feet in it.

Phytocil Powder A dusting powder containing zinc undeconoate, plus chlorophenoxyethanol and phenoxypropanol. Apply twice daily to feet, socks and the insides of shoes.

Quinoped A cream containing benzoyl peroxide plus potassium hydroxyquinoline sulphate. Massage into the affected area twice daily; then wash hands.

Scholl's Athlete's Foot Cream A white cream containing the long-established anti-fungal, tolnaftate. Apply twice daily.

Scholl's Athlete's Foot Powder A powder containing tolnaftate. Apply twice daily as **treatment** and once daily **to keep the infection away**.

Scholl's Athlete's Foot Solution An aerosol spray containing tolnaftate. Apply twice daily.

Tinaderm Cream containing the anti-fungal ingredient, tolnaftate. Apply twice daily.

Tinaderm Plus Powder Powder containing the anti-fungal tolnaftate. Shake between toes twice daily, and also into socks and shoes.

Tinaderm Plus Powder Aerosol Also contains tolnaftate (*see* above). Apply twice daily, and spray into shoes and socks.

Tineafax Powder A powder containing the anti-fungal, tolnaftate. Sprinkle on to feet, inside socks and inside shoes twice daily.

Trosyl Dermal Cream Contains 1% ticonazole (an anti-fungal). Apply twice daily.

Valpeda Cream containing halquinol. Useful against athlete's foot and some other infections as well. Apply night and morning, after washing and drying feet thoroughly.

Whitfield's Ointment Excellent traditional remedy, unfortunately no longer available in some countries. Invented by British dermatologist Dr Whitfield, it contains compound benzoic acid. Highly effective against athlete's foot, it is fierce stuff, so do not be tempted to apply it to anywhere but the feet. Keep well away from the eyes.

COLDS

GENERAL ADVICE
Before you start spending money on any remedies, it is important to realise that there is NO cure for colds. No antibiotic, prescription drug or proprietary cold remedy will cure it – or indeed shorten it.

All you can do is try things that will ease the symptoms. There is no point in going to your doctor and asking him to prescribe something for you; it makes far more sense to use a remedy from your local chemist's. The pharmacist will usually be more than willing to hear what your symptoms are, and suggest a product which could make them more bearable.These are listed below.

But do bear in mind that some people think they have a cold when in reality they have something else. A cold is confined to your head. It produces the following symptoms:

* sneezing
* a runny nose

* a blocked-up feeling
* runny eyes
* a general sense of being decidedly 'under the weather'

If you have other symptoms, such as a cough, earache or breathlessness, you have more than a cold and should seek professional advice.

Also, a cold should only last for about seven days. If you have symptoms which have gone on for much longer than this, it is **not** a cold that you have. See your doctor and get yourself checked out.

*(See also the sections on **Coughs**, **Flu** and **Sore Throats**).*

WARNING

1 Many of the preparations in this section contain either aspirin or paracetamol. Overdose of either can be FATAL. So be very wary about taking more than one type of cold remedy on the same day.

2 You will find that many of the remedies listed contain a 'decongestant'. If you have high blood pressure or heart problems, avoid taking such products by mouth. They can also react badly with certain anti-depressants.

3 Many of the products also contain a 'sedative anti-histamine'. These drugs can make you drowsy or even put you to sleep. Do **not** take them if you are going to drive, or operate machinery or computers. You should also avoid alcohol when taking these products.

Over-the-counter preparations for colds include:

Actifed Syrup Contains two drugs which 'decongest' the upper air passages. Do not use if you have high blood pressure or heart trouble.

Can cause problems with certain anti-depressant drugs. Follow pharmacist's advice carefully.

Actifed Tablets Same ingredients as Actifed Syrup *(see* above*)* and same warnings apply. Good for unblocking air passages.

Afrazine Nose drops with active ingredient oxymetazoline. Used for clearing blocked noses, but do not use for more than a few days. Take pharmacist's advice about possible interactions with other drugs.

Aspirin Excellent remedy for cold symptoms, but do not exceed 12 tablets a day, and **do not give to children**. Also, do not take if you are breast-feeding, have an ulcer, or are aspirin-sensitive. Take great care if you have asthma, as this drug may cause you to wheeze.

Beechams Hot Blackcurrant Sachets containing paracetamol *(see* warnings under **Paracetamol**, later in this section*)*, vitamin C and phenylephrine, plus blackcurrant flavouring. Phenylephrine is a decongestant that should be avoided if you have heart trouble or high blood pressure. It may also interact with some antidepressants – so seek a pharmacist's advice.

Beechams Hot Lemon Sachets of powder with the same ingredients as Beechams Hot Blackcurrant *(see* above*)*, but flavoured with lemon instead of with blackcurrant.

Beechams Hot Lemon & Honey Sachets with the same ingredients as Beechams Hot Lemon, but flavoured with lemon and honey.

Beechams Powders Traditional remedy containing caffeine (the mild stimulant in coffee), plus the equivalent of two aspirin tablets *(see* warnings under **Aspirin**, above*)*.

Beechams Powders Capsules Unlike Beechams Powders *(see* above*)*, these contain paracetamol (in place of aspirin) *(see* warnings under ***Paracetamol***, later in this section*)*. The capsules also contain caffeine, plus the same decongestant as in Beechams Hot Blackcurrant *(see* previous page*)*.

Benylin Day & Night Comes as a pack of yellow and blue tablets. The yellow tablets contain paracetamol *(see* warnings under ***Paracetamol***, later in this section*)* plus a decongestant. The blue ones contain paracetamol plus a sedative anti-histamine.

Catarrh-Ex Capsules containing a small dose of caffeine (as a stimulant), plus paracetamol *(see* warnings under ***Paracetamol***, later in this section*)* and a decongestant.

Coldrex Tablets containing caffeine, paracetamol *(see* warnings under ***Paracetamol***, later in this section*)*, vitamin C, terpin (which can cause tummy upsets), and a decongestant.

Coldrex Powders Blackcurrant-flavoured powders containing paracetamol *(see* warnings under ***Paracetamol***, later in this section*)*, vitamin C, and a decongestant.

Contac 400 Capsules containing a sedative anti-histamine, and a decongestant.

Day Nurse Capsules Orange and yellow capsules containing paracetamol *(see* warnings under ***Paracetamol***, later in this section*)*, a decongestant and dextromethorphan, a mild cough suppressant which can make you slightly constipated.

Day Nurse Liquid Same ingredients as Day Nurse Capsules *(see* above*)*.

Dristan Spray Nose spray containing the decongestant oxymetazoline, plus camphor, menthol

and eucalyptus. Do not use this product for more
than a week.

Dristan Tablets Quite different from Dristan Spray
(see above*).* White/yellow tablets containing
caffeine (the mild stimulant in coffee), plus a
decongestant, and the sedative anti-histamine,
diphenylpyraline.

Eskornade Syrup Syrup containing the same drugs
as Dristan Tablets *(see* above*),* in slightly different
proportions.

Fenox Nasal spray or nose drops – both containing
the decongestant phenylephrine. Do not use for
more than a week.

Flurex Capsules Capsules containing paracetamol
(see warnings under ***Paracetamol***, later in this
section*)* and a decongestant, plus the mild cough
suppressant dextromethorphan, which may cause
slight constipation.

Flurex Tablets Pink tablets containing paracetamol
(see warnings under ***Paracetamol***, later in this
section*),* the mild stimulant caffeine, and the
decongestant phenylephrine.

Friar's Balsam Popular traditional remedy –
reassuring and with little risk of side-effects.
Contains aloes plus prepared storax and sumatra
benzoin, and 90% alcohol.

Karvol Decongestant capsules. Contents can be
sprinkled on bedding (avoid skin contact), or added
to hot water for inhalation. Main ingredients include
cinnamon, pine and menthol. Natural and soothing.

Lemsip Powder containing the equivalent of 1.3
paracetamol tablets *(see* warnings under
Paracetamol, later in this section*),* plus vitamin C
and the decongestant phenylephrine.

Lemsip Cold Relief Capsules Capsules containing caffeine (the mild stimulant in coffee, plus three-fifths of a paracetamol tablet *(see* warnings under **Paracetamol**, opposite*)* and the same decongestant as in Lemsip *(see* previous page*)*.

Lemsip Junior Powder intended for children: contains rather less than half a paracetamol tablet *(see* warnings under **Paracetamol**, opposite*)*, plus a small amount of vitamin C, a decongestant and some sodium citrate.

Lemsip Menthol Extra Powder containing the same ingredients as Lemsip *(see* previous page*)*, but with the addition of menthol vapours.

Lemsip Night Time Liquid containing the equivalent of one and one-fifth paracetamol tablets *(see* warnings under **Paracetamol**, opposite*)*, a sedative anti-histamine, a decongestant, a cough suppressant (dextromethorphan, which may cause constipation), and alcohol. **Not suitable for children.**

Mackenzies Smelling Salts Ammonia and eucalyptus-containing smelling salts, intended to relieve catarrh.

Mentholatum Vapour Rub Traditional-style remedy that can either be rubbed into the chest and neck and the fumes breathed in, or else put in a bowl of hot water and inhaled. Contains menthol, camphor and methyl salicylate.

MuCron Tablets Contains the equivalent of one paracetamol tablet *(see* warnings under **Paracetamol**, opposite*)*, plus a decongestant.

Night Cold Comfort Capsules Capsules containing the equivalent of three-fifths of a paracetamol tablet *(see* warnings under **Paracetamol**, opposite*)*, plus a decongestant, a sedative anti-histamine, and a mild cough suppressant.

Night Nurse Capsules Contain the equivalent of one paracetamol tablet (*see* warnings under **Paracetamol**, below), plus a sedative anti-histamine and the mild cough suppressant dextromethorphan, which may cause slight constipation. Designed to be taken at bedtime.

Night Nurse Liquid Syrup containing paracetamol (*see* warnings under **Paracetamol**, below), a sedative anti-histamine, and the mild cough suppressant dextromethorphan, which may cause slight constipation. To be taken at bedtime.

Nosor Nose Balm Soothing nose application, containing various traditional ingredients such as camphor, menthol, eucalyptus and wheatgerm oil.

Olbas Oil Popular remedy for congestion, designed to be inhaled from a handkerchief or pillow, or from hot water. Contains various natural products, such as cajuput oil.

Olbas Oil Pastilles Pastilles containing various natural oils, plus menthol. To be sucked.

Otrivine Nasal Drops (Adult Formula) Contain the decongestant xylometazoline. Do not use for more than a week.

Otrivine Nasal Spray Contain the same ingredients as Otrivine Nasal Drops (*see* above). Do not use for more than a week.

Paracetamol Much used for the relief of cold symptoms. Overdosage (more than eight tablets a day) may damage the liver and can even prove fatal. Many cold remedies contain paracetamol – so do not take paracetamol tablets at the same time.

Penetrol Catarrh Lozenges Soothing lozenges containing menthol, creosote, ammonium chloride and a decongestant.

Penetrol Inhalant Intended to be inhaled from a handkerchief. Contains menthol and peppermint oil.

Sinutab Nightime Tablets Pink tablets containing the equivalent of three-fifths of a paracetamol tablet (*see* warnings under **Paracetamol**, on previous page), plus a decongestant and phenyltoloxamine (mildly sedative).

Sinutab Tablets Similar to Sinutab Nightime Tablets (*see above*), but without the mildly sedative ingredient, so can be taken during the day.

Sudafed Elixir Elixir containing the decongestant pseudoephedrine (*see* **Warning** above).

Sudafed Tablets Decongestant tablets containing the same ingredient as Sudafed Elixir (*see* above).

Sudafed-Co Tablets Same ingredient as Sudafed Tablets (*see* above), plus the equivalent of one paracetamol tablet (*see* warnings under **Paracetamol**, on previous page).

Throaties Catarrh Pastilles Contain traditional ingredients, including menthol, honey and lemon oil.

Tixylix Inhalant Children's remedy, to be sprinkled on to pillow or into hot water for inhalation. Contains menthol and other traditional inhalants.

Triogesic Tablets Contain the equivalent of one paracetamol tablet (*see* warnings under **Paracetamol**, on previous page), plus a decongestant.

Triominic Tablets containing a decongestant (phenylpropanolamine) plus a sedative anti-histamine.

Vapex Designed to be inhaled from a handkerchief or tissue. Contains the traditional remedy, menthol.

Vicks Cold Care Capsules containing the equivalent of slightly more than three-fifths of a paracetamol tablet *(see* warnings under **Paracetamol**, earlier in this section*)*, plus a decongestant and a mild cough suppressant.

Vicks Inhaler Traditional 'anti-blockage' sniffer, containing camphor and menthol.

Vicks Medinite Syrup containing paracetamol *(see* warnings under **Paracetamol**, earlier in this section*)*, a decongestant, a mild cough suppressant (which may cause slight constipation) and doxylamine (slightly sedative). For bedtime use only.

Vicks Sinex Nasal spray. Contains menthol and a eucalyptus derivative, plus oxymetazoline. Do not use for more than a week.

Vicks VapoRub Traditional-style remedy, designed to be rubbed on the chest or added to hot water, and inhaled.

Wright's Vaporizing Fluid An inhalant containing the traditional remedy chlorocresol. Must be used with a special vaporiser. ***Not suitable for children under 3***.

COLD SORES

GENERAL ADVICE
Cold sores do not have anything to do with colds. They are blistery eruptions on the lip, caused by the herpes simplex virus. Sufferers often get a 'warning' in the form of a tingly sensation in the lips before an attack.

It is thought that the virus is usually picked up during childhood when a youngster is kissed by an infected adult. Unfortunately, the virus then 'hibernates' inside the nervous system, occasionally flaring up and causing a cold sore.

During an attack, you should not kiss anybody or touch them with your face, and you should most **definitely not** have oral sex, in case you spread the virus to your partner's genitals.

If you are a parent, you should try hard to avoid any unnecessary physical contact with your children while you have a cold sore on your lip. If you can delegate such activities as bathing the children to your partner, so much the better.

During attacks, wash your hands frequently. Do not share towels with others; use disposable tissues for drying yourself, and put them in a plastic rubbish bag afterwards.

NOTE: If you can 'diagnose' very early on that you are getting a cold sore — ideally at the 'tingly' stage before the sore is visible – then it is well worth buying Zovirax Cold Sore Cream *(see* below*)* and applying it.

Over-the-counter preparations for cold sores include:

Blisteze Cream A cream containing ammonia and phenol. Apply every hour.

Brush Off Cold Sore Treatment An antiseptic paint containing povidone iodine. Do not use if you are sensitive to iodine.

Lypsyl Cold Sore Gel An anaesthetic and antiseptic ointment. The local anaesthetic can cause a sensitivity reaction in some people.

Zovirax Cold Sore Cream Start using as early as possible during an attack. Apply five times daily for five days.

CONSTIPATION

GENERAL ADVICE
There is a good deal of confusion about medication for constipation. Most doctors are not particularly keen on over-the-counter constipation remedies, and would much rather that you simply ate a lot more fibre-containing foods, such as fruit, vegetables, cereals and wholemeal bread, and also bran.

These 'natural remedies' are now preferred, because it is felt that our Western diet has been too low in fibre for a long time. Also, doctors are concerned about the long-term effects of laxatives: they can interfere with the absorption of essential nutrients and, in some cases, they can also cause low blood potassium levels.

Please note that excessive use of laxatives can lead to a situation where the bowel more or less gives up functioning altogether.

Furthermore, before buying an anti-constipation product, you should ask yourself 'Am I really constipated?' A lot of people think they are simply because they do not have a bowel action every day. Nowadays, doctors do not believe that it is essential to have a daily bowel action; there are some healthy people who 'go' only once every two or three days – though there are others who pass motions several times a day.

Finally, all adults should bear one thing in mind. If you have a sudden and unexplained change in bowel habit (such as constipation), **_you must get yourself checked out by a doctor_**. This is particularly important if you are over the age of 40.

So if that happens to you, do not treat yourself blindly with a constipation remedy; instead, seek medical advice.

CLASSES OF LAXATIVES

* Bulk-forming laxatives (such as ispaghula husk, sterculia, and methyl cellulose) can cause wind and tummy discomfort

* Faecal softeners (such as paraffin) make passing stools easier, but can cause anal irritation and other side-effects

* Osmotic laxatives (such as magnesium sulphate, lactulose and sodium compounds) work by 'sucking' fluid into the bowel. Do not take any sodium-containing products if you have heart, kidney or liver problems

* Irritant laxatives can cause colicky pain and (with long-term use) a 'non-functioning bowel'. They include phenolphthalein, senna and aloin. Phenolphthalein can cause rashes and discolouration of the urine

Over-the-counter preparations for constipation include:

Agarol Emulsion containing agar, liquid paraffin and phenolphthalein.

Alophen Pills containing phenolphthalein and aloin.

Andrews Liver Salts Popular, traditional remedy, containing bicarbonate of soda, citric acid and magnesium sulphate.

Beecham's Pills Famous old remedy that contains aloin.

Bonomint Laxative chewing gum, containing phenolphthalein.

Brooklax Tablets Chocolate bar containing phenolphthalein.

Califig The well-known California Syrup of Figs, containing extract of senna.

Calsalettes Tablets containing aloin; available in sugar-coated and non sugar-coated forms.

Carters Little Pills Long-established brand of pills containing phenolphthalein and aloin.

Celevac Pink pills containing the bulk-forming laxative methyl cellulose.

Correctol Contain phenolphthalein and dioctyl sodium sulphosuccinate.

Dulco-lax Suppositories Contain bisacodyl.

Dulco-lax Tablets Tablets containing the same ingredient as Dulco-lax Suppositories *(see* above*)*.

Duphalac Yellow solution containing lactulose and related carbohydrates.

Ex-lax Chocolate Tablets Chocolate tablets containing phenolphthalein.

Ex-lax Pills Pills containing an almost identical amount of phenolphthalein to Ex-lax Chocolate Tablets *(see* above*)*.

Fybogel and Fybogel Orange Sachets of granules containing ispaghula husk.

Fybranta Chewable tablets containing bran and calcium phosphate.

Isogel Granules Brownish-red granules of ispaghula husk.

Juno Junipah Salts Old remedy containing sodium sulphate, phosphate and bicarbonate, and also juniper oil.

Juno Junipah Tablets Tablets containing sodium sulphate, phosphate and chloride, plus juniper oil and phenolphthalein.

Kest White tablets containing magnesium sulphate plus phenolphthalein.

Laxoberal Yellow liquid containing sodium picosulphate.

Manevac Sugar-coated granules containing the fibrous seed of the plantago plant, plus senna.

Metamucil A bulk-forming laxative containing ispaghula husk.

Milk of Magnesia Traditional old remedy: white fluid containing magnesium hydroxide.

Milk of Magnesia Tablets Tablets containing the same ingredient as milk of Magnesia *(see* above*)*.

Mil-par White liquid, containing magnesium hydroxide plus liquid paraffin.

Normacol Granules containing sterculia.

Nylax Red tablets containing phenolphthalein, senna and bisacodyl.

Petrolagar No 1 Thick white mixture of petrolagar.

Proctofibe Tablets containing fibrous extracts of citrus and grain.

Regulan Powder containing ispaghula husk, flavoured with lemon and lime, or orange.

Reguletts Chocolate-flavoured tablets containing phenolphthalein.

Regulose Liquid containing lactulose.

Senlax Chocolate bar containing senna.

Senokot Granules Long-established remedy
containing senna in granule form.

Senokot Syrup A syrup version of Senokot Granules
(see above).

Senokot Tablets Senna-containing tablets.

SureLax Raspberry-flavoured chewable tablets,
containing phenolphthalein.

COUGHS

GENERAL ADVICE

The vital point to grasp about a cough is this. **It is
happening for some reason**. That is why doctors are
reluctant to give you drugs to 'suppress' a cough –
they would much rather diagnose the cause.
Unfortunately, in most countries it is very easy to
buy cough suppressants, but a good pharmacist will
try and direct you away from purchasing such a
product if she thinks that simply suppressing the
cough will do no good.

However, it **is** justifiable to buy yourself a cough
suppressant if you have a dry, irritating cough that
is keeping you awake at night.

WARNING: You MUST go to a doctor if:

* you cough up blood, or rusty-coloured sputum

* you are bringing up green or yellow sputum
   (phlegm) – this indicates that you have an
   infection, which may need antibiotic treatment

* your cough goes on for more than a week (this
   is especially important if you are a smoker)

* you experience pain or breathlessness

* your child's cough is persistant – this may indicate asthma, so she or he needs a check-up as soon as possible.

The main types of cough medicine available fall into the following groups:

COUGH SUPPRESSANTS These are drugs that numb the 'cough control' centres in the brain. As mentioned above, they should only be used as a short-term measure to 'damp down' a dry, irritating cough that is keeping you awake at night. Drugs in this group include codeine, dextromethorphan and pholcodine.

DECONGESTANTS These should not be taken by anyone with heart trouble or high blood pressure. They may interact with certain anti-depressants – ask your pharmacist's advice.

EXPECTORANTS These are medicines that are supposed to help you cough things up. Most doctors are very doubtful that they do anything at all – but they are still popular. They include ipecacuanha, squills and ammonium chloride. Some medicines contain both an expectorant and a suppressant.

DEMULCENTS These are 'soothing' preparations that many people take to try and relieve a dry, irritant cough. Again, doctors are doubtful if they have any real value, but some patients swear by them. They include sugary and non-sugary syrups, and glycerol.

ANTI-HISTAMINES These are of value if there is an allergic element in the cough, but probably not otherwise. They produce sedation, and this undoubtedly makes some people feel better. DO NOT DRINK, DRIVE OR OPERATE MACHINERY IF YOU ARE ON AN ANTI-HISTAMINE PREPARATION.

NOTE: If you have a cough, do not smoke, and keep away from other people who smoke.

Over-the-counter preparations for coughs include:

Actifed Compound Linctus Contains a cough suppressant, an anti-histamine, and a decongestant. For dry, tickly coughs.

Actifed Expectorant Contains a decongestant, an anti-histamine, and an expectorant. Intended for 'chesty' coughs.

Actifed Junior Cough Relief Contains a cough suppressant and an anti-histamine. Sugar-free.

Balm of Gilead Cough Mixture Old-fashioned herbal remedy containing tinctures of squills and lobelia, plus balm of gilead liquid extract.

Balm of Gilead Pastilles Not the same as Balm of Gilead Cough Mixture *(see* above*)*. Contain only an extract of bud of gilead.

Beecham Coughcaps Capsules containing tiny 'beads', each of which contains the cough suppressant dextromethorphan. For dry coughs.

Benylin Chesty Cough Linctus (Original) Red syrup containing menthol plus a sedative anti-histamine.

Benylin Chesty Coughs (Non-Drowsy) A raspberry-flavoured syrup containing an expectorant and some menthol. Will not make you drowsy.

Benylin Dry Coughs (Original) Raspberry-flavoured liquid containing a cough suppressant and a sedative anti-histamine.

Benylin Dry Coughs (Non-Drowsy) Peach-flavoured syrup containing the cough suppressant dextromethorphan only. No sedative, so will not make you drowsy.

Benylin Childrens Coughs (Original) Red syrup containing menthol and a sedative anti-histamine.

Benylin Children's Coughs (Sugar-Free; Colour-Free) Syrup containing menthol and a sedative anti-histamine, but with no added sugar or colouring.

Benylin with Codeine Red syrup containing a cough suppressant (codeine) plus a sedative anti-histamine and some menthol.

Bronalin Dry Cough Syrup containing a decongestant and a cough suppressant in alcohol. Sugar-free; colour-free.

Bronalin Expectorant Contains an expectorant and a sedative anti-histamine. Said to make coughs 'more productive'.

Buttercup Syrup Blackcurrant-flavoured liquid containing an expectorant, plus menthol and the sugar, glucose.

Buttercup Syrup (Honey & Lemon) Very similar formula to Buttercup Syrup *(see above)*, but with a third of a gramme of honey per teaspoonful.

Buttercup Lozenges Soothing lozenges containing bee propolis. Available in honey and lemon flavours or blackcurrant.

Cabdriver's Cough Linctus Imaginatively-titled old remedy containing a cough suppressant, plus various natural oils and terpin (which can cause tummy upsets).

Cabdriver's Junior Linctus Contains a decongestant, an expectorant, glucose and red poppy syrup.

Cabdriver's Sugar-Free Linctus Formula designed to be suitable for diabetics.

Copholco Cough Syrup Contains a cough suppressant, plus menthol, cineole, and terpin (which can cause tummy upset). Intended for dry, ticklish coughs.

Copholcoids Cough pastilles containing the same ingredients Copholoco Cough Syrup *(see above)*, but in different proportions. Also for dry, ticklish coughs.

Cupal Baby Cough Syrup Blackcurrant-flavoured syrup containing dilute acetic acid. Said to soothe irritating coughs in children aged over three months.

Davenol Linctus Tangerine/orange-flavoured liquid containing a decongestant, a cough suppressant and an anti-histamine.

Dimotane Expectorant Contains a decongestant, an expectorant and a sedative anti-histamine.

Dimotane Co (Dimotane With Codeine) Contains a cough suppressant (codeine), plus a decongestant and a sedative anti-histamine. Intended for coughs with colds.

DoDo Expectorant Linctus Brown liquid containing the expectorant guaiphenesin.

DoDo Tablets with totally different composition from DoDo Expectorant Linctus *(see above)*. Contain caffeine (the mild stimulant in coffee) plus a decongestant and the anti-wheeze drug theophylline.

Famel Expectorant Contains the expectorant guaiphenesin. Intended for the relief of 'tight, chesty coughs'.

Famel Linctus Contains the cough suppressant pholcodeine. For the relief of 'dry, tickly coughs'.

Famel Original Syrup containing creosote, plus a cough suppressant (codeine phosphate).

Famel Pastilles Lemon and honey-flavoured cough pastilles containing the expectorant guaiphenesin.

Fisherman's Friend Honey Cough Syrup Traditional remedy containing honey, squill vinegar, and various natural oils.

Franolyn for Dry Coughs Yellow liquid containing the cough suppressant dextromethorphan.

Hill's Balsam Adult Expectorant Brown mixture containing the expectorant guaiphenesin.

Hill's Balsam Adult Suppressant Brown mixture containing the cough suppressant pholcodine.

Hill's Balsam Pastilles Contain an expectorant plus menthol, peppermint oil, benzoin tincture and capsicum.

Jackson's All Fours Syrup containing the expectorant guaiphenesin.

Lemsip Chesty Cough Linctus containing the expectorant guaiphenesin.

Lemsip Dry Tickly Cough Soothing linctus, containing only honey, glycerin and citric acid.

Liqufruta Blackcurrant-flavoured liquid, containing menthol, glucose and an expectorant.

Meltus Expectorant Liquid containing sugar, honey, an expectorant, and the antiseptic cetylpyridinium. Intended for chesty coughs.

Meltus Cough Linctus Contains the expectorant guaiphenesin, plus honey and lemon flavouring.

Meltus Dry Cough Elixir Liquid containing the cough suppressant dextromethorphan.

Owbridge's (Chesty Coughs) Liquid containing the expectorant guaiphenesin.

Owbridge's (Dry, Tickly and Allergic Coughs) Liquid containing the cough suppressant dextro-methorphan, plus glycerin.

Phensedyl Plus Contains a sedative anti-histamine, plus a decongestant and a cough suppressant.

Pholcodine Linctus which suppresses dry or painful cough. Possible side-effects include constipation.

Robitussin For Chesty Coughs Contains the expectorant guaiphenesin.

Robitussin For Chesty Coughs With Congestion Contains the expectorant guaiphenesin, plus a decongestant (pseudoephedrine).

Robitussin For Dry Coughs Contains the cough suppressant dextromethorphan.

Sudafed Expectorant Contains the expectorant guaiphenesin, plus a decongestant.

Sudafed Linctus Contains the cough suppressant dextrmethorphan, plus the same decongestant as in Sudafed Expectorant *(see above)*.

Tancolin Children's Linctus Contains the cough suppressant dextromethorphan, plus vitamin C.

Throaties Family Cough Linctus Traditional-style remedy containing honey, lemon oil and other mild ingredients, plus an expectorant.

Throaties Pastilles Fruit-flavoured menthol and eucalyptus pastilles.

Tixylix Daytime For dry coughs in children. Contains the suppressant pholcodine.

Tixylix Nighttime Blackcurrant linctus containing the suppressant pholcodine, plus a sedative anti-histamine.

Vegetable Cough Remover Imaginatively-titled traditional-style remedy containing at least 17 very mild ingredients, including horehound and skunk cabbage.

Veno's for Dry Coughs Syrup containing only glucose and treacle. Will not make you drowsy.

Veno's Expectorant for Chesty Coughs Contains glucose and treacle plus an expectorant. Will not make you drowsy.

Veno's Honey and Lemon for Tickly Coughs Glucose, honey and lemon juice only. No drugs.

Vicks Original Formula Cough Syrup Expectorant Contains guaiphenesin expectorant, plus sodium citrate and cetylpyridinium, an antiseptic.

Vicks VapoSyrup for Chesty Coughs Contains the expectorant guaiphenesin, in higher doses than Vicks Original Formula Cough Syrup Expectorant *(see* above).

Vicks VapoSyrup for Chesty Coughs and Nasal Congestion Like Vicks VapoSyrup for Chesty Coughs *(see* above), but also contains a decongestant.

Vicks VapoSyrup for Dry Coughs Contains the suppressant dextromethorphan.

Vicks VapoSyrup for Dry Coughs and Nasal Congeston Like Vicks VapoSyrup for Dry Coughs *(see above),* but with a decongestant as well.

CYSTITIS

GENERAL ADVICE
Cystitis is very common problem indeed. The main symptoms are:

* pain on passing water
* having to keep rushing to pass water
* sometimes, blood in the urine

Many cases are the result of germs getting into the bladder and causing inflammation. Most commonly these are germs that live in the bowel, which are thought to have crossed the short distance from the anus to the urinary opening.

In a lot of other cases, tests do not reveal any infection in the urine. It is possible that in some of these, the attack of cystitis is caused by germs which standard laboratory tests do not detect.

However, many bouts of cystitis seem to be caused simply by sexual activity which – particularly in the case of young, inexperienced couples – may cause minor trauma round the urinary pipe (hence the expression 'honeymoon cystitis').

If you get an attack of cystitis you should go to your GP, who should send a carefully-collected specimen of your urine to the laboratory for analysis **before** giving you any antibiotics.

However, if you are unable to get to a doctor, the Kilmartin self-help regime for emergency treatment of cystitis may relieve symptoms. It is popular in British Commonwealth countries and, to a lesser extent, France. Proceed as follows:

1 Take a pain-killer (aspirin or paracetamol)

2 Drink plenty of water

3 Take sodium bicarbonate to try to make the urine less acid (unless you are on a low salt diet)

4 Place a hot water-bottle on the lower tummy, and another between the thighs. Contact a doctor within 48 hours if there is no improvement.

Several of the products listed below are also intended to make the urine less acid. Again, avoid those that contain sodium bicarbonate if you are on a low-salt diet. Those that contain potassium may cause stomach irritation.

Over-the-counter preparations for cystitis include:

Cymalon Granules containing sodium bicarbonate, plus two other sodium compounds and citric acid.

Cystemme Granules containing sodium citrate.

Cystoleve Powder containing sodium citrate.

Cystopurin Powder containing potassium citrate.

Effercitrate Fizzy tablets containing potassium bicarbonate and citric acid.

Potter's Antitis A herbal remedy containing several plant extracts, including buchu leaf.

DIARRHOEA

GENERAL ADVICE
There are many over-the-counter products available for treating diarrhoea.

However, there are a number of circumstances in which you should NOT attempt to treat yourself or your family, but should call in a doctor instead.

These circumstances include:

* If you are living in or passing through a region where really serious causes of diarrhoea are common (such as a tropical country)

* If you have just come back from a holiday abroad

* If a bout of diarrhoea is making you feel very ill

* If the diarrhoea has gone on for more than about two days and is not improving

Most important of all: if a young child has diarrhoea, **do not attempt to treat it yourself**.

Babies and toddlers can rapidly become very seriously ill if they have a bad bout of diarrhoea. So it is important to get medical advice without delay. You should also bear in mind that most attacks of diarrhoea, especially those which 'go round' a family, are caused by infection. Therefore, it is vital that if anyone in a household has diarrhoea, everybody should take great care about hygiene. In particular:

* Make sure everyone washes their hands after going to the toilet

* Hands should also be washed before eating, and before preparing food.

How do you choose which over-the-counter remedy to buy if somebody in your family gets diarrhoea? Doctors tend to favour 'rehydrating' preparations, designed to replace the vital minerals lost during an attack of diarrhoea. In contrast, members of the public often want pills or medicines which will **stop** the diarrhoea. To be honest, this is rarely possible.

If you get an attack of diarrhoea, my advice is to avoid eating for 24 hours, drink plenty of water, and buy one of the 'rehydrating' preparations listed below. If you also want to take something to try and stop the diarrhoea, then choose from the preparations listed here. If still in doubt about choice of brand, seek advice from your pharmacist.

NOTE: You will see that many 'diarrhoea-stoppers' contain the drug loperamide. This can cause tummy-ache, a bloated feeling, and skin reactions. The British Consumers' Association has recently claimed that it can make you retain toxic materials in the bowel, though this remains a subject of controversy. ***Do not give it to children under 12.***

Over-the-counter preparations for diarrhoea include:

Arret Capsules containing 2 mg of loperamide.

Collis Browne's Mixture Old remedy containing peppermint oil, chloroform water and a very small dose of morphine (too much of this can cause vomiting and drowsiness).

Collis Browne's Tablets Tablets containing kaolin, calcium carbonate and a small amount of morphine (can cause nausea/drowsiness).

Diareze Capsules containing 2 mg of loperamide.

Diocalm Dual Action Contains a small dose of morphine (can cause nausea/drowsiness), plus attapulgite – an absorbent.

Diocalm Replenish A well-balanced rehydration formula.

Diocalm Ultra Different from other Diocalm products (see above): contains 2 mg of loperamide.

Dioralyte Blackcurrant A well-balanced rehydration formula in fizzy tablet form, with blackcurrant flavour.

Dioralyte Plain Sachets of powder containing well-balanced rehydration formula. Available in citrus or blackcurrant flavours.

Electrolade Well-balanced rehydration formula. Available in banana or melon flavours.

Enterosan Tablets containing kaolin, belladonna and a small dose of morphine (excess can cause nausea/drowsiness).

Glucolyte Sachets containing well-balanced rehydration formula in powder form.

Imodium Capsules containing 2 mg of loperamide.

Kaolin and Morphine Mixture (Mist. Kaolin et Morph.) Traditional remedy. The morphine can cause nausea/drowsiness, and dependence may occur after repeated use.

Opazimes Tablets containing morphine (may cause nausea/drowsiness), aluminium hydroxide, belladonna and kaolin.

Rapolyte Raspberry-flavoured powder containing a well-balanced rehydration formula.

Rehidrat Well-balanced rehydration formula, flavoured with orange, lemon or lime.

EAR TROUBLES

GENERAL ADVICE
Ears are delicate things, so I do **not** recommend that you put anything inside them unless it is on medical advice.

There is one exception to this rule. If you know that your ears are partly blocked with wax, then it is perfectly all right to soften it up (and, with luck, dissolve it away completely) with one of the 'anti-ear wax' products listed below, or olive oil. However, solid and tenacious wax will probably need removing by a doctor or trained nurse.

WARNING: Always contact a doctor in cases of:

* earache
* discharge from the ear
* bleeding from inside the ear
* unexplained deafness
* unexplained noises in the ear

You should **never** attempt to treat any of the above symptoms yourself and, in particular, do not poke anything inside the ear, or block it up with cotton wool.

Over-the-counter preparations for ear troubles include:

Audax Drops for softening ear wax. Also marketed for relief of ear pain, but do **not** use them for this until you have been examined by a doctor.

Cerumol Ear drops for loosening wax.

Dioctyl Ear Drops Solution for softening and loosening ear wax.

Earex Ear drops for softening and loosening wax.

Exterol Solution for softening and loosening wax.

Molcer Drops for softening and loosening wax. Also marketed for the relief of earache, but do **not** use for this purpose until you have first been examined by a doctor.

Otex Squeeze bottle containing drops for softening ear wax.

Waxsol Drops to aid wax removal; use on no more than two consecutive nights before syringing by a doctor or nurse.

Waxwane Drops (delivered from dropper) for softening wax prior to medical syringing.

EYE TROUBLES

GENERAL ADVICE

Your eyes are among the most delicate parts of your body, so NEVER put anything in them unless you are really sure that you know what you are doing. Take special care to read the label – immediately before use – because it is extremely easy to pick up the wrong thing and put it in your eyes by mistake. (Contact lens wearers should take particular note of this warning – it is not uncommon for people to accidentally put lens cleaner or disinfectant in the eye, instead of eye drops.)

Most of the preparations in this section are for minor irritations of the eye – for instance, those caused by dust. But I do stress the word 'minor'.

You MUST consult a doctor if you have any of the following:

* a red, angry-looking eye
* a sticky eye – in other words, one that is producing yellowish-coloured stuff
* pain in the eye
* difficulty in seeing
* a foreign body in the eye – unless it is just a little fleck that can be removed with the corner of a clean handkerchief.

Contact lens wearers frequently have special problems with their eyes. If in the slightest doubt about any symptom, contact your contact lens practitioner or a doctor. Remember also that some over-the-counter eye preparations may stain your lenses; as a general rule, do not put anything in your eye while wearing your lenses unless your practitioner has told you it is safe to do so.

Over-the-counter preparations for eye troubles include:

Brolene Soothing drops containing propamidine. If no improvement after two days, see a doctor.

Brolene Eye Ointment Ointment containing an ingredient similar to that in Brolene *(see above)*. If no improvement after two days, see a doctor.

Eye Dew Intended to give clearer whites. Contains witch hazel plus a drug (naphazoline) which you should **not** use if you have glaucoma or other serious eye problems.

Hypotears For temporary relief of minor discomfort and 'dry eyes'.

Isopto Alkaline Colourless tear replacement solution.

Isopto Frin Quite different from Isopto Alkaline *(see above)*, intended for minor irritation. Contains an ingredient (phenylephrine) which must not be used in cases of eye disease, after eye surgery, or if you have high blood pressure.

Isopto Plain Tear replacement solution, similar to Isopto Alkaline *(see above)* but a different strength.

Lacrilube Lubricating eye ointment. Use only under professional direction.

Liquifilm Preservative-Free For same purpose as Liquifilm Tears *(see next entry)*. Contains povidone – do not use if sensitive to this.

Liquifilm Tears Artificial tears for dry eyes.

Minims Artificial Tears Single-use ampoules for those with insufficient tears. May cause blurring when first put in.

Minims Sodium Chloride Colourless salt solution for irrigating the eye. Suitable for use with contact lenses.

Murine Anti-redness drops. Contain naphazoline – do **not** use if you have glaucoma or other serious eye problems.

Optrex Well-known traditional eye lotion containing distilled witch hazel; apply using eye bath. Also available as drops (with boric acid and borax).

Optrex Clearine Eye drops containing witch hazel and naphazoline – which must not be used if you have glaucoma or other serious eye conditions. Diminishes redness of whites.

Otrivine-Antistin Drops for relief of redness and itching due to allergies, etc. Contain xylometazoline and antazoline. If you have any eye or medical disorders, check with doctor before using.

Sno Tears Colourless artificial tears for dry eyes.

Sooth-eye Drops Eye drops containing zinc sulphate. For minor irritation. May sting slightly.

Tears Naturale Artificial tear fluid for dry eyes.

FLU

GENERAL ADVICE
Influenza (flu) is only common during the flu epidemics which sweep across the world every now

and then. However, there are millions of people who claim to have flu – and sincerely believe that they have it – when they are only suffering from a cold, or some other virus infection.

Real influenza usually gives the following symptoms:

* a high temperature
* feeling terrible
* aches and pains all over

There may also be 'cold-like' symptoms such as sneezing, a blocked nose or a sore throat.

How do you tell the difference between a cold and an attack of the flu? A wise doctor once said that if you feel well enough to cross the road and pick up a fifty dollar note lying in the gutter, you probably just have a cold. If you don't, you probably have flu.

But if you think you may have flu, then the best thing to do is ring your doctor and ask for advice. This is especially important if you are elderly, or have heart, chest or kidney trouble – because flu can often be very serious for those who are already not too well.

Unfortunately, penicillin and other antibiotics have no effect at all on flu (though doctors sometimes prescribe them in order to combat 'secondary' infections which have developed while the body is weakened by influenza). So – just as with a cold – all you can do is to treat the symptoms until recovery occurs, which usually takes about a week.

Good ways of treating the symptoms are:

* staying in bed
* drinking plenty of fluids
* using any of the popular pain killers/fever relievers: aspirin, paracetamol or ibuprofen (*see* entries later in this section)

You can also try one of the proprietary products listed in this section. But take great care not to choose one containing aspirin or paracetamol if you have already taken a dose of either drug.

Alcohol, in moderation, can also ease flu symptoms. In my view, a single whisky is probably of as much value as many proprietary remedies.

Over-the-counter preparations for flu include:

Aspirin As good an anything for flu. But do not use if you have an ulcer, or are sensitive to aspirin. Can cause wheezing in asthmatics. ***Do not give to children under 12.***

Beechams Hot Lemon Paracetamol-containing. For details, *see* section on ***Colds***.

Beechams Powders Aspirin-containing. For details, *see* section on ***Colds***.

Benylin Day & Night Paracetamol-containing. For details, *see* section on ***Colds***.

CatarrhEx Paracetamol-containing. For details, *see* section on ***Colds***.

Day Nurse Capsules Paracetamol-containing. For details, *see* section on ***Colds***.

Day Nurse Liquid Paracetamol-containing. For details, *see* section on ***Colds***.

Eskornade Spansules Relieves nasal congestion. For details, *see* section on ***Colds***.

Eskornade Syrup Relieves nasal congestion. For details, *see* section on ***Colds***.

Flurex Cold/Flu Capsules Paracetamol-containing. For details, *see* section on ***Colds***.

Flurex Tablets Paracetamol-containing. For details, *see* section on **Colds**.

Ibuprofen Like aspirin and paracetamol, ibuprofen is a useful standby for flu, because it relieves aches and pains, and helps lower temperature. Widely marketed under the brand name Nurofen. Do **not** take if you have an ulcer, or are sensitive to aspirin or any of the other common pain-relieving drugs. Drugs of this group may make asthma worse. Although this drug has been around for many years, it has not been used as widely as aspirin or paracetamol, and it is possible that there could be side-effects that have not yet been recognised.

Lemsip Paracetamol-containing. For details, *see* section on **Colds**.

Lemsip 'Flu Strength Contains more paracetamol than Lemsip *(see* above*)*, plus vitamin C, and a decongestant (avoid if you have high blood pressure or heart problems; may also react with certain anti-depressants).

Lemsip Menthol Extra Paracetamol-containing. For details, *see* section on **Colds**.

Lemsip Night Time Paracetamol-containing. For details, *see* section on **Colds**.

Mucron Tablets Paracetamol-containing. For details, *see* section on **Colds**.

Night Cold Comfort Tablets Paracetamol-containing. For details, *see* section on **Colds**.

Night Nurse Cold & 'Flu Remedy Capsules Paracetamol-containing capsules. For details, *see* section on **Colds**.

Night Nurse Liquid Paracetamol-containing. For details, *see* section on **Colds**.

Olbas Oil Soothing inhalant. For details, *see* section on *Colds*.

Olbas Oil Pastilles Soothing pastilles. For details, *see* section on *Colds*.

Paracetamol Useful in easing aches and pains and lowering temperature. But beware: do **not** exceed the stated maximum of eight 500 mg tablets per day. Please note that many other flu remedies contain paracetamol, so do not take any of them at the same time as paracetamol tablets. Paracetamol can occasionally cause skin rashes, blood disorders and pancreas problems. Even a small overdose may cause potentially fatal liver damage.

Sinutab Nightime Tablets Contain paracetamol plus a sedative anti-histamine. For details, *see* section on *Colds*.

Sinutab Tablets Paracetamol-containing. For details, *see* section on *Colds*.

Sudafed Co Contain paracetamol plus the same decongestant as in Sudafed Tablets *(see* below*)*. For details, *see* section on *Colds*.

Sudafed Elixir Contains a decongestant. For details, *see section on* *Colds*.

Sudafed Tablets Contain the decongestant pseudoephedrine; do not take if you have high blood pressure or heart trouble.

Uniflu with Gregovite C Tablets Contain paracetamol *(see* warnings under *Paracetamol*, above*)*, codeine phosphate (which can cause slight constipation), diphenhydramine (a sedative anti-histamine), phenylephrine (a decongestant – so do not take if you have high blood pressure or heart trouble), plus caffeine (the mild stimulant in coffee), plus vitamin C.

Vicks Cold Care Despite the name, will also help with flu symptoms. Paracetamol-containing. For details, *see* section on ***Colds***.

HAY FEVER AND OTHER NOSE ALLERGIES

GENERAL ADVICE
Apart from hay fever, there are various other nasal allergies – including the very common allergy to the droppings of the house-dust mite. In all these conditions, simple common-sense measures can greatly lessen the need for drugs.

HAY FEVER In Europe and certain other parts of the world, hay fever is caused by allergy to grass pollen. In the USA, the principal – but not the only – cause of hay fever is allergy to ragweed pollen.

Sensible practical measures to combat hay fever include the following:

* Staying indoors on days when the pollen count is high (these are usually warm, dry days)

* Having net curtains on open windows

* Keeping your car windows rolled up

* Wearing 'wrap-around' sunglasses

* Wearing an anti-pollution nose mask

* If possible, going to areas where pollen counts tend to be lower (eg the seaside).

OTHER NASAL ALLERGIES Once the cause of the allergy has been identified, there are a number of practical measures you can take in order to avoid the 'allergen'.

For instance, if you are allergic to the droppings of the house-dust mite, you can cut down your exposure to it by getting rid of as many dusty furnishings and hangings as possible, and enclosing your mattress in a special protective cover.

MEDICAL TREATMENT People who have hay fever or any other nasal allergy should begin by going to their GP. He may suggest anti-histamines or prescription only nasal applications. These modern treatments are highly effective. Do **not** take over-the-counter drugs as well unless your doctor says it is safe to do so.

However, these is a place for self-medication with over-the-counter drugs, especially when you are familiar with your own allergy well, and know what will control it.

WARNING: Remedies which contain sedative anti-histamines will probably make you drowsy. So do not drive, drink alcohol, or operate machinery or computers.

Nasal decongestant nose drops should not be used for more than a week at most. If taken by mouth, decongestants should not be used by people with high blood pressure or heart trouble. They may react very badly with certain types of anti-depressant.

Over-the-counter preparations for hay fever and other nose allergies include:

Actifed Tablets Tablets containing a sedative anti-histamine (triprolidine) and a decongestant (pseudoephedrine).

Actifed Syrup Syrup containing the same ingredients as Actifed Tablets *(see above)*.

Afrazine Nose spray containing the decongestant oxymetazoline. Do not use for more than a week.

Aller-eze Plus Tablets containing the sedative anti-histamine clemestine, plus a decongestant (phenylpropanolamine).

Aller-eze Tablets Contain a larger dose of the same sedative anti-histamine as Aller-eze Plus *(see above)*.

Beconase Hayfever Very useful anti-allergy nose spray containing a mild steroid (beclomethasone). Unfortunately, many people use it the wrong way. It is of no value in treating attacks; it has to be used twice daily, every day, in order to build up protection against 'allergens'.

Contac 400 Capsules containing a sedative anti-histamine (chlorpheniramine) plus the decongestant phenylpropanolamine.

Daneral SA Tablets containing a sedative anti-histamine (pheniramine).

Dimotapp Elixir Contains a sedative anti-histamine (brompheniramine), plus two decongestants (phenyl-propanolamine and phenylephrine).

Dimotapp LA Tablets Contain the same drugs as Dimotapp Elixir *(see above)*, in exactly the same proportions.

Dristan Spray Nose spray containing the decongestant oxymetazoline, plus camphor, menthol and eucalyptus.

Dristan Tablets Completely different from Dristan Spray *(see above)*. Contain a sedative anti-histamine (chlorpheniramine) and a decongestant (phenyl-ephrine), plus aspirin and caffeine (the mild stimulant in coffee).

Eskornade Spansules Sustained-release capsules containing a sedative anti-histamine (diphenyl-pyraline) plus a decongestant (phenyl-propanolamine).

Eskornade Syrup Greengage-flavoured syrup containing the same two drugs as Eskornade Spansules *(see* above*)* in very slightly different proportions.

Fenox Nose drops containing the decongestant phenylephrine. Do not use for more than a week.

Fenox Spray Nose spray containing the same ingredient as Fenox *(see* above*)*. Do not use for more than a week.

Haymine Sustained-release tablets containing a sedative anti-histamine (chlorpheniramine) plus a decongestant (ephedrine).

Hismanal Tablets containing one of the newer (and much less sedative) anti-histamines, astemizole. There is a small risk of heart problems with this drug, so never exceed the stated dose and do **not** take with other drugs. At present, banned in pregnancy; avoid conception for several weeks after taking it.

Histryl Spansules Sustained-release capsules containing the sedative ant-ihistamine, diphenylpyraline.

One-A-Day Antihistamine Tablets Contain the newer and much less sedative anti-histamine, terfenadine. This occasionally causes hair loss. It also carries a small risk of heart problems, so do not exceed the stated dose or take with other drugs.

Opticrom Allergy Eye Drops Contain sodium cromoglycate – a long-established anti-allergy agent. Useful for treating the eye symptoms of hay fever, but must be used regularly; there is no point in trying to treat attacks with the drops. Note: if symptoms persist, consult your doctor.

Otrivine-Antistin Eye drops containing antazoline and xylometazoline. They relieve redness and itching, but see doctor if symptoms persist.

Otrivine Hay Fever Formula Nasal Drops Nose drops containing the same two drugs as Otrivine-Antistin *(see above)*. Do not use this product for more than one week.

Penetrol Contains various agreeably-scented natural oils. Intended to be sniffed from a handkerchief. Keep away from eyes.

Phenergan Well-known blue tablets containing the sedative anti-histamine, promethazine.

Piriton Yellowish tablets containing the well-known, but sedative anti-histamine, chlorpheniramine.

Piriton Syrup Syrup containing the same drug as Piriton *(see above)*.

Pollon-Eze Tablets containing astemizole. For details and important warnings, *(see **Hismanal** on previous page)*.

Resiston One Nasal Spray Contains the decongestant xylometazoline, so do not use for more than a week. Also contains the anti-allergy drug cromoglycate which is ideally to be used long-term.

Rynacrom Compound Nasal solution containing the anti-allergy protector cromoglycate, with the decongestant xylometazoline.

Rynacrom Nasal Spray containing the anti-allergy protector cromoglycate. Should be used on a long-term basis.

Rynacrom Nasal Drops Contain the same drug as Rynacrom Nasal Spray *(see* opposite*)*.

Seldane Tablets containing terfenadine. For details and important warnings, *see **One-A-Day Antihistamine Tablets**,* earlier in this section.

Tavegil Tablets containing the sedative anti-histamine, clemastine.

Tavegil Syrup Syrup containing the same drug asTavegil *(see* above*)*.

Triludan Tablets containing 60 mg of terfenadine. For details and important warnings, *see **One-A-Day Anti-histamine Tablets**,* earlier in this section.

Triludan Forte Tablets containing the same drug as Triludan *(see* above*)*, but at twice the strength.

Triominic Yellow tablets containing the sedative anti-histamine pheniramine, plus the decongestant phenylpropanolamine.

Zirtek Contains the newer and much less sedating anti-histamine, cetirizine. Do not take if you have kidney problems, except on medical advice.

HEAD LICE

GENERAL ADVICE
The first thing to say about head lice is that catching them is not due to any lack of hygiene and is nobody's fault. People feel great embarrassment about having lice, but there really is no justification for it.

The second important point to make about head lice is this: if one member of the family catches them, you should treat every member of the family, since there is a high chance that brothers and sisters and Mum and Dad may be infected too. Failure to do this will quite often lead to the condition breaking out again.

If you find that one or more of your children has head lice, you should ask your GP or another health professional which of the many available anti-lice preparations you should use.

It is difficult for the non-medical person to make an informed choice – especially as there is now a considerable problem with resistance. In other words, some strains of lice have become resistant to certain drugs.

In Britain and some other countries, health authorities tend to operate special schemes to try and combat the problem of resistance. They rotate the choice of drugs that are used in the district, so that Drug A is used for a period of time, then Drug B for a while, and so on.

If this is the case in your area, then it makes sense to follow your local policy about choice of drug, rather than picking one of your own.

Good agents for dealing with head lice are malathion and carbaryl. They are available as lotions and shampoos. While shampoos are more pleasant to use, they have the disadvantage of not being in contact with the parasites for very long – so that they may not be killed. Doctors now tend to recommend having the anti-lice drug on the scalp for about 12 hours.

Whatever treatment you use, I recommend that you repeat it after a week, just to make certain that the 'nits' have all gone.

NOTE: Some anti-lice preparations contain alcohol, which is highly inflammable. So do **not** use a hair dryer after application. Preparations containing alcohol can affect asthmatic people adversely.

Over-the-counter preparations for head lice include:

Carylderm Lotion Alcohol-based lotion containing carbaryl 0.5%.

Carylderm Shampoo Contains carbaryl 1%.

Clinicide Lotion Liquid containing carbaryl 0.5%.

DerbacC Liquid Blue liquid containing carbaryl 1%.

DerbacC Shampoo Yellow shampoo containing carbaryl 0.5%.

Full Marks Lotion Alcohol-based lotion containing phenothrin 0.2%.

Lyclear Creme Rinse Rinse containing permethrin 5% (can cause itching, stinging or redness).

Prioderm Lotion Alcoholic solution containing malathion 0.5%.

Prioderm Shampoo Cream shampoo containing malathion 1%.

Rapell Alcoholic solution containing 2% piperonal, which is described as a hair lice repellent. Use with caution, if you have asthma or sensitive skin.

Suleo-C Lotion Alcohol-based lotion containing 0.5% carbaryl.

Suleo-C Shampoo Green shampoo containing 0.5% carbaryl.

Suleo-M Lotion Alcohol-based containing 0.5% malathion.

INDIGESTION

GENERAL ADVICE

The trouble with the word 'indigestion' is people use it to mean many different things. Its meaning varies wildly not only from person to person, but also from country to country. As far as this book is concerned, we are going to assume that if you say you have indigestion, you mean that you have one or more of the following common symptoms:

* Pain in the upper part of the abdomen (the 'tummy' or 'belly')

* Discomfort or a 'blown out' feeling in the same region – often accompanied by belching

The most important thing to realise is that these symptoms – particularly pain – can have serious causes. So you should **not** 'self-treat' yourself for very long. If indigestion persists for more than a week, you should go and get yourself examined by your doctor.

There is a huge variety of indigestion remedies available over-the-counter. Some of them are mild but virtually all of them can have side-effects, so take special care to read the label and any instructions enclosed with the remedy. You should also follow any directions the pharmacist gives you.

POWERFUL ANTI-ULCER DRUGS In the last few years, some countries have allowed over-the-counter sales of certain of the potent anti-ulcer drugs (such as Zantac, Tagamet and Pepcid) previously available only on doctor's prescription. Make sure you read the information given below on their side-effects.

SODIUM COMPOUNDS Indigestion remedies that contain sodium are best avoided if you are on a low-salt diet or have kidney problems.

HYOSCINE Remedies that contain this drug must be avoided if you have glaucoma.

ALUMINIUM COMPOUNDS Remedies containing aluminium may sometimes cause sickness and/or constipation.

MAGNESIUM COMPOUNDS Remedies containing magnesium may cause loose bowel motions. Avoid these remedies if you know that you have low blood phosphate levels.

BISMUTH COMPOUNDS Indigestion remedies containing bismuth may cause constipation.

CALCIUM COMPOUNDS Remedies containing calcium are best taken short-term only, as they can interfere with the body's mineral balance.

WARNING: Do *not* take 'antacids' with other drugs, as the antacid may interfere with them.

Over-the-counter preparations for indigestion include:

Actal Tablets White tablets containing sodium alexitol, an antacid.

Actonorm Powder Peppermint-flavoured powder containing compounds of sodium, aluminium, magnesium and calcium, plus atropine (avoid this remedy if you are elderly, or have glaucoma or prostate problems).

Actonorm Gel Contains aluminium and magnesium compounds, plus peppermint and dimethicone, an 'anti-wind' ingredient.

Alka-Seltzer Famous remedy containing sodium bicarbonate, citric acid and aspirin. However, the aspirin can sometimes irritate your stomach, rather than soothe it.

Alu-cap Aluminium hydroxide gel, inside a green/red capsule.

Aludrox Liquid Peppermint-flavoured gel containing aluminium hydroxide and aluminium oxide.

Aludrox Tablets Aluminium hydroxide, plus two magnesium compounds.

Andrews Antacid Chewable tablets containing calcium and magnesium carbonates. Also available in fruit flavour.

Andrews Liver Salts Sodium bicarbonate and magnesium sulphate. Acts as a laxative as well as an antacid.

Asilone Liquid Minty liquid containing magnesium oxide and aluminium hydroxide, plus the 'anti-wind' ingredient dimethicone.

Asilone Suspension Thick, mint and aniseed-flavoured, sugar-free liquid, containing the same ingredients as Asilone Liquid *(see above)*.

Asilone Tablets Contain aluminium hydroxide, plus the 'anti-wind' ingredient dimethicone.

Bicarbonate of Soda Traditional remedy, much valued by some people because it fizzes, and therefore causes belching. Best avoided if you have liver, kidney or heart problems, or are elderly.

Birley Antacid Powder Contains aluminium hydroxide, plus two magnesium compounds.

Bismag Tablets containing bicarbonate of soda *(see above)*, plus two varieties of magnesium carbonate.

BiSoDol Extra Tablets containing bicarbonate of soda *(see* above*)*, plus calcium carbonate and magnesium carbonate, and also the 'anti-wind' ingredient dimethicone.

BiSoDol Powder Contains bicarbonate of soda *(see* opposite*),* plus two varieties of magnesium carbonate.

BiSoDol Tablets Chewable. Contain bicarbonate of soda *(see* opposite*),* plus calcium carbonate and magnesium carbonate.

De Witt's Antacid Powder Contains bicarbonate of soda *(see* opposite*),* magnesium and calcium carbonates, magnesium trisilicate, plus kaolin and peppermint oil.

De Witt's Antacid Tablet Contain calcium and magnesium carbonate, plus magnesium trisilicate and peppermint oil.

Dijex Liquid Pink liquid containing aluminium hydroxide paste, plus magnesium hydroxide.

Dijex Tablets Chewable. Contain aluminium hydroxide and magnesium carbonate.

Double Action Indigestion Tablets Contain two antacids (aluminium hydroxide and magnesium hydroxide) plus the 'anti-wind' ingredient dimethicone.

Eno White fizzy powder containing bicarbonate of soda *(see* opposite*),* plus citric acid and sodium carbonate.

Gaviscon Liquid Fennel-flavoured liquid, containing bicarbonate of soda *(see* opposite*),* plus calcium carbonate and sodium alginate.

Gaviscon Tablets Contain bicarbonate of soda *(see* opposite*),* aluminium hydroxide, magnesium trisilicate, and alginic acid.

Gelusil Chewable/suckable tablets. Contain magnesium trisilicate and aluminium hydroxide.

Kolanticon Gel Contains aluminium hydroxide and magnesium oxide, plus the 'anti-wind' ingredient dimethicone, and the anti-spasm drug dicyclomine.

Maalox Plus Suspension Contains aluminium and magnesium hydroxides, plus the 'anti-wind' ingredient dimethicone.

Maalox Plus Tablets Contains the same ingredients as Maalox Plus Suspension *(see* above*).*

Maalox Suspension Contains aluminium and magnesium hydroxides.

Maclean Indigestion Tablets Minty tablets containing aluminium hydroxide, plus magnesium and calcium carbonates.

Milk of Magnesia Liquid Long-established remedy containing magnesium hydroxide. Laxative as well as antacid.

Milk of Magnesia Tablets Same ingredient as Milk of Magnesia *(see* above*).*

Moorland Tablets Contain calcium and magnesium carbonates, aluminium hydroxide, magnesium trisilicate and kaolin, plus bismuth aluminate, which may cause constipation.

Mucogel Suspension Contains aluminium and magnesium hydroxides.

Novasil Plus Suspension Contains aluminium and magnesium hydroxides, plus the 'anti-wind' ingredient dimethicone.

Nulacin Tablets containing calcium and magnesium carbonates, plus whole milk, dextrin and maltose.

Pepcid AC Tablets Contain famotidine, one of the powerful anti-ulcer drugs which have recently been made available without prescription in some countries. You can use Pepcid AC for **short-term** relief of indigestion, but you are advised not to continue it for more than two weeks without having your symptoms assessed by a doctor. Possible side-effects include dizziness, drowsiness and a rash.

PeptoBismol Suspension containing bismuth salicylate. Do not take this product if you are on aspirin or anticoagulants, or if you have gout. May make motions dark.

Remegel Chewy tablets containing calcium carbonate only.

Rennie (Digestif Rennie) Old-established tablets containing calcium and magnesium carbonates.

Rennie Gold Minty tablets containing calcium carbonate only.

Rennie Rap-Eze Contain a rather smaller dose of calcium carbonate than Rennie Gold *(see* above*)*, plus fruit flavouring.

Setlers Tablets containing calcium carbonate plus peppermint flavouring.

Setlers Tums Tablets containing calcium carbonate plus assorted fruit flavours.

Tagamet Contains cimetidine, which is one of the powerful anti-ulcer drugs recently made available without prescription in some countries. It is very effective for **short-term** relief of indigestion symptoms, but I advise you not to use it for more than two weeks without having your symptoms assessed by a doctor. Side-effects may include alteration in bowel habits, rash, dizziness, tiredness, confusion, headache, liver damage and (rarely) nipple enlargement and impotence. For more details, ask your pharmacist or doctor.

Windcheaters Imaginatively-named capsules which contain the well-known anti-gas ingredient dimethicone.

Zantac The brand name of ranitidine, another of the powerful anti-ulcer drugs (like Tagamet and Pepcid AC) which have recently been made more widely available to the public. Zantac is extremely effective at combatting acid, but I advise you not to use it for more than two weeks without consulting your doctor about your symptoms, and possible side-effects of the drug. Such side-effects could include alteration in bowel habits, rashes, dizziness, tiredness, confusion, liver damage and (rarely) nipple swelling and tenderness in men. If in doubt, ask your pharmacist or doctor.

PAINKILLERS (TAKEN BY MOUTH)

GENERAL ADVICE
Pain is all too common in life, so it is not really surprising that people buy vast quantities of pills intended to relieve it. It is also possible to ease pain using medications that are rubbed into the skin (*see* next section).

You will find that most of the pain-relieving products listed here contain one or more of the following three drugs:

* aspirin
* paracetamol
* ibuprofen (more widely known under the brand name Nurofen)

These three painkillers have been available for many years, though ibuprofen is newer than the other two. People have grown used to having them around, and often do not realise that they are powerful drugs which can have serious side-effects. So please read the warning notes below very carefully.

Most doctors favour 'ordinary' aspirin or 'ordinary' paracetamol over the branded products that contain them. Ordinary aspirin and paracetamol are also cheaper than branded products.

WARNINGS

* ASPIRIN is very good for headaches and muscular and 'rheumatic' pains. Do **not** take it for tummy ache, because the drug can irritate the stomach and make things worse. Do **not** take if you have ulcers. Aspirin can also cause bleeding from the stomach, wheezing (which can sometimes make it hazardous for asthmatic people), skin reactions, and problems with blood clotting. It can also react badly with certain drugs. **Not to be taken by children under 12**.

* PARACETAMOL is good for a variety of pains, and does not irritate the stomach. However, it can occasionally cause rashes, and blood and pancreas problems. Most importantly, it is easy to overdose accidentally on paracetamol, and this may cause severe or even fatal liver damage. Never exceed the stated dose of any paracetamol-containing product, or 8 tablets in 24 hours.

* IBUPROFEN, like aspirin, can irritate the stomach. It must not be taken if you have an ulcer, or a history of hypersensitivity to aspirin or any 'anti-rheumatic' drug, and especially if any of that group of drugs have made you wheeze. Excessive amounts can cause sickness, dizziness, drowsiness and incoordination. If you have asthma, check with your doctor before taking

ibuprofen. *Not suitable for children under the age of 12*.

Over-the-counter painkillers (taken by mouth) include:

Actron Contains both paracetamol and aspirin, plus fizzy ingredients and a dose of caffeine (the mild stimulant in coffee).

Alvedon PR Paracetamol suppositories.

Anadin Caplets Capsule-shaped tablets containing slightly more than one ordinary aspirin tablet, plus a small dose of caffeine.

Anadin Extra Capsules containing the equivalent of one aspirin and three-fifths of a paracetamol, plus a dose of caffeine.

Anadin Extra Soluble Soluble tablets containing the same pain-relieving ingredients as Anadin Extra *(see above)*.

Anadin Ibuprofen Tablets Completely different from all other Anadin products *(see above and below)*; contain ibuprofen only.

Anadin Maximum Strength Contain one and two-thirds of an aspirin, plus some caffeine.

Anadin Paracetamol Contain the equivalent of one paracetamol tablet.

Anadin Soluble Contain just over one aspirin, plus caffeine, in fizzy form.

Anadin Tablets Contain just over one aspirin, a tiny amount of quinine, and a small dose of caffeine.

Aspro Clear Contain the equivalent of one aspirin tablet, in soluble form.

Aspro Tablets Each contains slightly more than one aspirin.

Beecham Aspirin Tablets containing the equvalent of a quarter of one aspirin tablet.

Beechams Powders For headaches, plus colds and flu. Contain the equivalent of two aspirins, plus a dose of caffeine.

Cafadol Contain the equivalent of one paracetamol tablet, plus caffeine.

Calpol Extra for Adults Tablets containing the equivalent of one paracetamol, plus a small dose of codeine phosphate (may cause mild constipation), and a little caffeine.

Calpol (and Sugar-Free Calpol) Infant Suspension Popular pain-relieving medicines for young children. The pain-killing ingredient is paracetamol.

Calpol Six Plus A stronger suspension of paracetamol than Calpol Infant Suspension *(see above)*, for children aged 6 to 12.

Caprin Contain slightly more than one aspirin, in a slow-release formulation. Do not chew.

Co-Codamol Each tablet contains one paracetemol *(see* paracetamol) plus a little codeine phosphate.

CodaMed Marketed for 'tension headache'. Each tablet contains rather less than one paracetamol, plus some codeine phosphate and caffeine.

Codanin Each tablet contains the equivalent of one paracetamol tablet, plus some codeine phosphate (may cause slight constipation).

Codis 500 Each soluble tablet contains the equivalent of one and two-thirds of an aspirin tablet, plus some codeine phosphate (which may cause slight constipation).

Cojene Marketed for 'rheumatic pain'. Each tablet contains one aspirin, plus some codeine phosphate (may cause slight constipation) and caffeine.

Cullen's Headache Powders Sachets, each containing the equivalent of two aspirin tablets, plus some caffeine and calcium phosphate, which may cause slight constipation.

Cuprofen Film-coated tablets containing ibuprofen .

Cuprofen Soluble A soluble version of Cuprofen

De Witt's Analgesic Pills 'Analgesic' means 'painkilling'. Each pill contains about two-thirds of a paracetamol, plus some caffeine.

Disprin Soluble tablets, each containing the equivalent of one aspirin.

Disprin Direct Chewable version of Disprin tablets.

Disprin Extra Soluble tablets, each containing the equivalent of one aspirin tablet, plus two-fifths of a paracetamol tablet.

Disprol Each tablet contains one paracetamol.

Doan's Extra Strength Backache Pills Khaki-coloured tablets, each containing rather less than a third of a paracetamol, plus sodium salicylate (a close relative of aspirin).

EP Tablets Each contains one paracetamol, plus a dose of caffeine and some codeine phosphate.

Fanalgic Each tablet contains one paracetamol.

Fanalgic Syrup A paracetamol syrup.

Feminax White capsule-shaped tablets, each containing one paracetamol, some codeine phosphate (may cause slight constipation), a dose of caffeine, and hyoscine (an anti-spasm drug).

Fynnon Calcium Aspirin Soluble tablets, each containing one and two-thirds of an aspirin, plus calcium carbonate.

Hedex Each capsule-shaped tablet contains one paracetamol.

Hedex Extra Advanced Hedex Formula Each tablet contains one paracetamol, plus a dose of caffeine.

Inoven Caplets Each contains 200 mg of ibuprofen.

Junior Disprol Soluble (fizzy) paracetamol tablets for children.

Laboprin Each tablet contains one aspirin, plus the aminoacid lysine.

Librofem Pink tablets, each contains 200 mg of ibuprofen.

Medised Blackcurrant-flavoured paracetamol suspension, which also contains the sedative anti-histamine promethazine. Causes drowsiness.

Nurofen Well-known brand name for ibuprofen 200 mg.

Nurofen Soluble Soluble version of Nurofen tablets *(see* above*)*.

Nurse Sykes' Powders Each contains rather more than half an aspirin, plus almost a quarter of a paracetamol and some caffeine.

Pacifene Sugar-coated tablets containing 200 mg of ibuprofen.

Pacifene Maximum Strength Contain double the dose of Pacifene *(see* previous page).

Panadeine Each tablet contains one paracetamol, plus some codeine phospate (which may cause slight constipation).

Panadol Capsules Same as Panadol Tablets *(see* below*)*, but in capsule form.

Panadol Extra Each tablet contains the equivalent of one paracetamol, plus a dose of caffeine.

Panadol Soluble Fizzy tablets, each containing one paracetamol.

Panadol Tablets Well-known brand name for paracetamol; each tablet contains one paracetamol.

Panadol Ultra Maximum Strength Formula Each tablet contains one paracetamol, plus some codeine phosphate (may cause mild constipation).

Panaleve Capsules Each contains one paracetamol, plus some caffeine.

Paracets Each contains one paracetamol. Available as capsules or tablets.

Paracodol Capsules Each contains one paracetamol, plus some codeine phosphate (may cause mild constipation).

Paracodol Soluble Tablets The same as Paracodol Capsules *(see* above*)*, in soluble form.

Paramol Tablets Each contains one paracetamol, plus some dihydrocodeine tartrate (may cause mild constipation).

Phensic Tablets Each contains slightly more than one aspirin, plus some caffeine.

Phor Pain Pink tablets, each containing 200 mg of ibuprofen. Also available in double strength.

Powerin Super Strength Pain Reliever Each tablet contains one aspirin and two-fifths of a paracetamol, plus some caffeine.

Proflex SR Sustained-release capsules, each containing 100 mg of ibuprofen.

Proflex Tablets Contain 200 mg of ibuprofen.

Propain Each tablet contains four-fifths of a paracetamol, plus some codeine phosphate (may cause mild constipation) and caffeine, and a sedative anti-histamine diphenhydramine (so do not drink, drive or operate machinery).

Solpadeine Capsules Each contains one paracetamol, plus some codeine phosphate (may cause mild constipation) and some caffeine.

Solpadeine Tablets Same content as Solpadeine Capsules *(see above)*.

Tramil Each capsule contains one paracetamol.

Veganin Each tablet contains half a paracetamol and appreciably less than one aspirin, plus a little codeine phosphate (may cause mild constipation).

PAINKILLERS (APPLIED TO SKIN)

GENERAL ADVICE
Always remember that pain means something. If the pain persists or is very bad, consult a doctor.
Having said that, there are many fairly minor pains

that you can ease by rubbing a painkiller into your
skin. These are mainly muscular and 'rheumatic'
aches and pains caused by bruising and trivial
sports injuries.

There are two main types of pain relievers you can
rub into your skin:

* Traditional-style applications: These increase the
  blood supply to the area, and also cause a mild
  irritation of the skin which helps 'blot out' pain.

* Anti-rheumatic drug applications: These have
  become available in the last few years. They are
  simply 'skin' versions of the drugs that are so
  widely used for 'rheumatic' disorders.

It is claimed that after they have been rubbed into
the skin, these pain relievers are absorbed deeply
enough to have an effect on the painful muscle or
joint, but this is still controversial. At present, the
authoritative British National Formulary says that
anti-rheumatic drug applications 'may provide some
slight relief of pain'.

WARNING: Do not apply any of the products in this
section to broken or inflamed skin. And if any rash
or other odd skin reaction develops, stop using the
application at once and consult your doctor. All
products in this section should be kept away from
the eyes, mouth, and intimate areas.

If you are sensitive to aspirin, do not use any
product which is described as containing salicylates
(relatives of aspirin).

**Over-the-counter painkillers that can be applied
to the skin include:**

Algesal Traditional-style application containing a
salicylate (related to aspirin). Lavender-scented
cream.

Algipan Traditional-style application. Well-known 'rub', much used by athletes.

Algipan Spray Traditional-style 'warming spray'.

Balmosa Traditional-style application. A white cream containing a salicylate (related to aspirin) and other warming ingredients. Also for unbroken chilblains.

Bayolin Traditional-style application. Cream containing a salicylate (related to aspirin) and other warming ingredients.

BN Liniment Traditional-style application. Emulsion for rubbing into painful joints, etc.

Cremalgin A traditional-style remedy. Balm containing a salicylate (related to aspirin) and other warming ingredients.

Deep Freeze An aerosol spray which eases pain by 'freezing', much used by sports coaches. Do not spray on face, head, neck, fingers, toes or intimate areas. Avoid use in confined space.

Deep Heat Extra Strength A traditional-style remedy containing methyl salicylate (related to aspirin) and menthol.

Deep Heat Massage Liniment Traditional-style remedy, containing similar ingredients to Deep Heat Extra Strength (see above).

Deep Heat Rub Traditional-style remedy containing similar ingredients to Deep Heat Extra Strength (see above), plus eucalyptus and turpentine oils.

Elliman's Embrocation Traditional-style application. A mixture of turpentine oil and acetic acid.

Fiery Jack Ointment Traditional-style application. A long-established 'rubbing ointment'.

Goddard's White Oil Embrocation Traditional-style application containing turpentine oil, acetic acid and ammonia.

Ibuleve Gel Anti-rheumatic drug application containing ibuprofen.

Ibuleve Sports Gel Same ingredient as Ibuleve Gel (*see* above), in laminated pump-action tube.

Menthol and Wintergreen Heat Rub Traditional-style application containing methyl salicylate (relative of aspirin) and other warming ingredients.

Movelat Cream and Gel Traditional-style application containing salicylate acid (relative of aspirin), plus mucopolysaccharide polysulphate.

Oruvail Gel Anti-rheumatic drug application containing ketoprofen.

PR Freeze Spray Aerosol spray that eases pain by 'freezing'. Do not spray on face, head, neck, fingers, toes or intimate areas. Avoid use in confined spaces.

PR Heat Spray Traditional-style application. A warming spray in aerosol form.

RadianB Heat Spray Traditional-style application containing salicylate acid and ammonium salicylate (relatives of aspirin), in spray form.

RadianB Muscle Lotion Contains the same ingredients as RadianB Heat Spray (*see* above), plus warming ingredients.

RadianB Muscle Rub Contains methyl salicylate (relative of aspirin), plus warming ingredients.

Ralgex Cream Traditional-style cream containing a salicylate (relative of aspirin), plus warming ingredients.

Ralgex Freeze Spray Aerosol that eases pain by
'freezing'. Ozone-friendly; no CFCs. Avoid face and
intimate areas. Do not use in enclosed places.

Ralgex Low Odour Spray Traditional-style warming
application in spray form. CFC-free. Contains a
salicylate (relative of aspirin).

Salonair Traditional-style warming spray that
contains two salicylates (relatives of aspirin) plus
warming ingredients.

Tiger Balm Ointment (Regular White) Popular in
the Far East; a traditional-style remedy containing
cajuput oil, menthol, camphor and clove oil. Makes
the skin feel cool after use.

Tiger Balm Ointment (Extra Strength Red) A
stronger version of Tiger Balm Ointment (Regular
White) *(see* above*)*, containing more menthol.

Transvasin Heat Rub Traditional-style application,
containing a salicylate (relative of aspirin), plus
warming ingredients.

PERIOD PROBLEMS AND
PREMENSTRUAL SYNDROME
(PMS)

GENERAL ADVICE
If you have period problems, it is best to consult
your doctor, rather than trying to treat them yourself.
These days, most menstrual difficulties can be
cured (or greatly helped) by treatment from a GP or,
if necessary, a gynaecologist.

However, once you have been carefully examined
and assessed by a doctor, there may be times when

you need some extra help from an over-the-counter product, especially the painkilling tablets listed in the section on *Painkillers (Taken By Mouth)*.

There are only a few other products available without prescription, as you will see from the shortness of this section. This reflects the fact that the treatment available from doctors these days is usually so good. So please do not hesitate to get skilled medical advice.

WARNING: If you decide to use one of the products listed here, please note the following:

* Vitamin B6 (pyridoxine) does seem to help some women with premenstrual syndrome, but excessive use can cause problems. Read the label and stick to the stated dose.

* Some of the preparations listed here contain the painkiller paracetamol. Although this is an effective drug, taking even a little more than the stated dose can be very dangerous.

* Do *not* take products containing ibuprofen (a popular painkiller) if you have ulcers; there are more details about this drug at the start of the section on *Painkillers (Taken By Mouth)*.

* Preparations containing codeine phosphate may make you slightly constipated.

Over-the-counter preparations for period problems and PMS include:

Benadon Tablets containing either 20 mg or 50 mg of vitamin B6 (pyridoxine), for premenstrual symptoms.

Complement Continus Sustained-release tablets containing 100 mg of vitamin B6 (pyridoxine) for premenstrual symptoms.

EP Tablets Pain-relieving tablets containing the equivalent of one paracetamol tablet, plus codeine phosphate (which may cause slight constipation) and a dose of caffeine (the mild stimulant found in coffee).

Feminax This tablet has been mistaken for a contraceptive in the past, because of its name. In fact it is a painkiller which also attempts to relieve spasm of the womb. It contains the equivalent of one paracetamol tablet, plus codeine phosphate (which may cause slight constipation), caffeine, and the anti-spasm drug hyoscine.

Librofem Each tablet contains 200 mg of the painkiller ibuprofen.

Spasmonal Intended to relieve menstrual cramps; contains the anti-spasm drug alverine citrate.

Woman Kind Tablets intended for PMS; each contains 25 mg of vitamin B6 (pyridoxine).

PILES

GENERAL ADVICE
As a doctor, the most important thing I can say to you about piles (haemorrhoids) is this: do not assume that you have piles just because you have problems with your anus.

In particular, do not assume that anal bleeding **must** be due to piles. It can have much more serious causes, especially in those over the age of about 35.

So if you have any 'bottom problems', please do not just buy a pile remedy over-the-counter and hope that all will be well. Go and see your GP and get yourself checked out. This should include an

examination of the inside of the rectum, which is
embarrassing but essential.

Finally, please remember that even if you have had
piles for years, it is possible to develop other (and
more serious) problems as well. So you must
consult a doctor urgently if you develop any of the
following symptoms:

* unexplained change in 'bowel habit' (such as
  suddenly getting constipation or loose motions)
* persistent abdominal (tummy) pain
* passing black or tarry motions
* passing a lot of mucus
* rectal bleeding even though your piles seem to
  be under control

WARNING: Some of the anti-pile products listed
here contain a local anaesthetic, intended to relieve
pain. But local anaesthetics can cause painful
sensitivity reactions in some people.

Over-the-counter preparations for piles include:

Anodesyn Ointment Contains a local anaesthetic,
plus allantoin, a soothing agent with astringent
properties.

Anodesyn Suppositories Contain the same
ingredients as Anodesyn Ointment *(see* above*)*.

Anusol Cream Bland, soothing ointment, containing
zinc and bismuth oxides, plus balsam of Peru.

Anusol Ointment Contains the same chemicals as
Anusol Cream *(see* above*)*, plus bismuth subgallate.
Being an ointment, this preparation will stay longer
on the skin than the cream will.

Anusol Suppositories Very soothing, bland
suppositories, containing the same chemicals as
the Anusol Ointment *(see* above*)*.

Dermidex Cream containing various ingredients, including a local anaesthetic.

Germoloids Cream Contains zinc oxide, plus a local anaesthetic ingredient.

Germoloids Ointment Contains the same ingredients as Germoloids Cream *(see* above*)*. Being an ointment, this preparation stays longer on the skin than the cream will.

Germoloids Suppositories Contain the same ingredients as Germoloids Cream and Ointment *(see* above*)*.

Heemex An old-established remedy containing various soothing ingredients; formulated to relieve itching.

Hemocane Cream containing various soothing ingredients plus a local anaesthetic.

Hemocane Suppositories Contain the same chemicals as Hemocane *(see* above*)*.

Lanacane Cream containing soothing ingredients plus a local anaesthetic.

Nupercainal A local anaesthetic cream.

Preparation H Ointment Unusual but time-honoured remedy containing only yeast cell extract and shark liver oil.

Preparation H Suppositories Contain the same ingredients found in Preparation H Ointment *(see* above*)*.

TCP Ointment Yellow antiseptic ointment containing a wide variety of ingredients, including iodine (do not use if sensitive to iodine). This preparation can cause staining of underwear.

SLEEPLESSNESS

GENERAL ADVICE
In the last few years, there has been a tendency for more 'sleep promoting' products to be sold without prescription. However, my medical advice to you is that if you are having real trouble in sleeping, you should **always** begin by consulting a doctor, because there is usually some reason for it.

Very frequently, sleeplessness is a symptom of an underlying depressive illness, which your GP can give you help with. There are also other causes of insomnia which need medical help.

Most of the sleeping pills which are now allowed on the market without prescription are sedative anti-histamines. Do not underestimate the potency of these drugs. You should bear the following in mind:

* You can get hooked on them

* People who come off them after a long period can sometimes suffer fits

* They can make you drowsy next day, with resulting bad effects on your driving skills or your ability to operate computers or machinery

* You must **not** drink alcohol while you are under their influence

IMPORTANT: If you suffer from one of the rare group of disorders called 'the porphyrias', do not take any of these drugs except on medical advice.

Over-the-counter remedies for sleeplessness include:

Boots Herbal Restful Night Tablets Contain the soothing herb passiflora. No anti-histamines.

Kalms Tablets Traditional herbal remedy, containing valerian, gentian and humulus. Does not contain anti-histamines.

Natracalm Herbal remedy containing passiflora. No anti-histamines.

Natrasleep Herbal tablet containing valarian and humulus. No anti-histamines.

Nytol Contains the anti-histamine diphenhydramine (which is also used in the popular cough and cold remedy, Benylin).

Passiflora (Gerard) Tablets containing the herb of the same name. No anti-histamines.

Phenergan Tablets Contain the sedative anti-histamine promethazine.

Sominex Tablets Contain the same anti-histamine as in Phenergan *(see above)*, but at twice the strength. Check label for details.

SMOKING REMEDIES

GENERAL ADVICE
Smoking is disastrous for many people's health, and if you smoke your life will probably be shortened. So it is well worth trying hard to give up.

Unfortunately, giving up is very difficult, mainly because nicotine (the drug in tobacco) is highly addictive. So if you go without it, you usually feel terrible to begin with.

It is really only willpower that can make you beat the craving, but moral support from your doctor, friends and family can often help, as can some of products listed in this section. The idea behind them is to give you a certain amount of the drug to keep you going as you learn to manage without cigarettes.

But the nicotine-containing products listed here are a long way from being 100 per cent effective. Indeed, most studies suggest that they help only a minority of smokers to give up. Be wary of the fact that it is quite easy to become dependent on the nicotine-containing product itself, and take care not to exceed the dose stated on the pack.

WARNING: Nicotine-containing products (including cigarettes) should **not** be used by anyone who has heart disease, high blood pressure, circulatory problems or a history of thrombosis (clots).

Do **not** use them if you are pregnant or breast-feeding, and do **not** combine them with other nicotine-containing products, which again includes cigarettes. Please note that nicotine patches may cause irritation of the skin.

Over-the -counter anti-smoking preparations include:

Nicabate Patches Nicotine-containing skin patches. The idea is to start with the 'strong' patches and gradually work down to the weak ones.

Nicobrevin Capsules containing eucalyptus oil, camphor, quinine and methyl valerate. It is claimed that they decrease your desire for tobacco.

Nicorette Chewing Gum Gum containing nicotine. Will certainly help a minority of smokers to give up.

Nicorette Patches Nicotine-containing skin patches that are used in a similar way to Nicabate Patches (*see* above).

Nicotinell Patch Programme Nicotine-containing skin patches used in a similar way to Nicabate and

Nicorette Patches *(see above)*. If you are a heavy smoker, you start with a stronger patch.

Stubit Lozenges containing nicotine.

SORE THROATS

GENERAL ADVICE
Sore throats are usually caused by one of the following three things:

1 Infections with viruses. These cannot be cured with penicillin or other antibiotics. All you can do is treat the symptoms with products like throat lozenges, and perhaps take aspirin or paracetamol.

2 Infections with bacteria. These are less common than infections with viruses. If your doctor suspects that you could have a bacterial infection, she may put you on an antibiotic. Throat lozenges and pastilles may be helpful in relieving the symptoms, and it may also be worth taking a painkiller, such as aspirin or paracetamol.

3 Smoking. Although they usually do not realise it, most smokers have a low-grade inflammation of the throat, so it is not surprising that it flares up from time to time. If you are a smoker and you get sore throats, the remedy is to give up smoking. However, some sore throats in smokers are due to a combination of smoke and infection.

WARNING: Some sore throat preparations contain the antiseptic chlorhexidine. This can stain your teeth permanently and can occasionally cause irritation of the mouth or throat.

Some products for sore throats contain local anaesthetics. These can sometimes cause painful sensitivity reactions. Do not use if you have had any previous adverse reactions to a local anaesthetic-containing product.

Over-the-counter preparations for sore throats include:

Bradosol Plus Lozenges containing the antiseptic domiphen, plus a local anaesthetic.

Bradosol Sugar Free Completely different to Bradosol Plus *(see* above*)*, containing only the antiseptic benzalkonium chloride.

Dequacaine Lozenges containing an antiseptic (dequalinium), plus a local anaesthetic.

Ernest Jackson's Antiseptic Throat Pastilles
Pastilles containing a combination of traditional antiseptics.

Labosept Pastilles Contain the antiseptic dequalinium.

Mac Extra Pleasantly flavoured lozenges, each containing the antiseptic hexlresorcinol.

Mentholatum Antiseptic Lozenges Flat lozenges containing menthol and eucalyptus oil, plus the antiseptic amylmetacresol.

Merocets Lozenges containing the antiseptic cetylpyridinium.

Merothol Lozenges containing eucalyptol, plus the antiseptic cetylpyridinium.

Merocaine Lozenges containing the antiseptic cetylpyridinium, plus a local anaesthetic.

Proctor's Pinelyptus Pastilles Contain four traditional remedies, including menthol and eucalyptus oil.

Strepsils Contain the antiseptics amylmetacresol and dichlorobenzyl alcohol. Also available with vitamin C.

TCP Pastilles Contain TCP liquid antiseptic plus flavouring. Available in blackcurrant, lemon or honey and menthol varieties.

Throaties Extra Contain three traditional remedies, including menthol.

Tyrocane Throat Lozenges Contain the antiseptic cetylpyridinium, plus the anti-infection agent tyrothricin, and a local anaesthetic.

Tyrozets Aniseed-flavoured lozenges, containing the anti-infection agent tyrothricin, plus a local anaesthetic.

Valda Pastilles Traditional remedy, containing a combination of five soothing ingredients, including menthol and thymol.

Vicks Ultra Chloraseptic Throat spray containing a local anaesthetic.

Zensyls Lime-flavoured lozenges, containing the antiseptic benzalkonium chloride.

THRUSH

GENERAL ADVICE
Vaginal thrush is one of the most common ailments of Western women. It is caused by a fungus, which many people carry in their bodies, and which tends to flare up from time to time.

The chief symptom is a white, irritant discharge (like cottage cheese in appearance), accompanied by redness, soreness and itching of the vaginal opening.

In recent years, it has become common to buy over-the-counter remedies for thrush. In my view, if you have the above symptoms **you should go to a doctor and have proper tests done.**

This is because thrush is quite easy to confuse with other conditions. Also, your doctor may be able to identify the factor that has made the thrush flare up. He will probably prescribe one of the anti-fungal creams mentioned in this section, plus anti-fungal pessaries (vaginal tablets).

If possible, your sexual partner should also use the anti-fungal cream, because otherwise there is a risk of the fungus continuing to be passed to and fro between you.

Your doctor will probably also recommend that you take the following common-sense anti-thrush measures during an attack:

* Avoid too many hot baths during an attack – have cool showers instead, but do not over-wash

* Wear stockings instead of tights

* Choose cool cotton pants instead of synthetic ones; if necessary, go without pants during an attack of thrush

If you have had previous attacks of thrush and, most importantly, have learned to recognise the symptoms with reasonable certainty, then it is perfectly acceptable to buy an over-the-counter product which will clear up the infection rapidly.

But if your symptoms **do not** clear up on over-the-counter self-treatment, then do go to your doctor for an examination and tests.

WARNING: Although it is unlikely that this will happen, anti-fungal drugs can occasionally provoke sensitivity reactions in some people. So if irritation gets worse instead of better, you should consult your doctor.

Over-the-counter preparations for thrush include:

Canesten 1 VT Vaginal tablets containing the anti-fungal clotrimazole. Best used with 1% Canesten Cream *(see* below) externally.

Canesten Cream 1% Contains the same ingredient as Canesten 1 VT *(see* above); for external use (i.e. on the vulva). Best combined with Canesten 1 VT vaginal tablets *(see* above).

Canesten 10% VC A stronger vaginal cream than Canesten Cream 1% *(see* above), but with the same ingredient; inserted high into the vagina at night using a special applicator (provided).

Femeron Cream containing the anti-fungal miconazole. Apply externally (i.e. to the vulva). Best used at the same time as Femeron Soft Pessaries *(see* below).

Femeron Soft Pessaries Egg-shaped vaginal capsules containing the same anti-fungal agent as Femeron cream *(see* above). Insert high into the vagina at night.

'TONICS'

GENERAL ADVICE
The public has always tended to believe in 'tonics'. Alas, any doctor will tell you that there is no such thing. So if you are not feeling terribly well, my advice is to go and see your doctor, talk to her about your symptoms, and if necessary have a thorough physical check-up. It could well be that your feelings are caused by a medical condition,

such as anaemia, depression, or a viral infection, for example.

So what are the products which are marketed as 'tonics'? For many generations manufacturers have produced potions that taste bitter, because this sort of taste is said to stimulate the appetite.

Other tonics have traditionally contained substantial amounts of alcohol. Be careful that you are not taking something that is giving you rather more drink than is good for you.

Iron is often included in 'tonics'. This will be of value if you are a victim of iron-deficiency anaemia, but not otherwise.

One final common ingredient of 'tonics' is glycerophosphate. I can only say that this chemical is not used in medical practice.

Over-the-counter 'tonics' include:

Effico Contains caffeine (the mild stimulant in coffee) and two vitamins of the B group.

Koladex Tablets Contain caffeine, plus dried extract of kola nut.

Labiton Contains 29% alcohol, plus some caffeine, vitamin B1, and dried extract of kola nuts.

Metatone Red liquid containing vitamin B1, plus four different types of glycerophosphate.

Minadex Tonic An orange-flavoured product which claims to 'build up children fast'. Can also be taken by adults. Contains vitamins A and D2, iron, copper, copper sulphate and two types of glycerophosphate.

Phyllosan Tablets containing a useful dose of iron, several B vitamins and a small dose of vitamin C.

Seven Seas Tonic Contains iron, vitamins A and D, copper and magnesium sulphates, and two kinds of glycerophosphate.

TRAVEL SICKNESS

GENERAL ADVICE

Many people – especially children – suffer from travel sickness. I recommend the following ways of dealing with it:

1 Don't keep talking to the (potential) victim about travel sickness or suggesting that he might be going to be sick

2 Distract him as much as possible during a journey. Children can be encouraged to look out of the window and to play 'I-spy', etc

3 Keep car windows open so that fresh air gets in

4 Don't smoke near the person

5 Don't give them a big meal just before setting out

6 Make sure you have a supply of plastic bags close at hand for the moment when a wavering voice says 'I feel sick'

Over-the-counter remedies can help, though they cannot work miracles. You must give them to the sufferer at least an hour before the journey starts. Dishing them out when the person is already feeling nauseated is probably too late.

There are two groups of travel sickness remedies: sedative anti-histamines and anti-spasm drugs.

Sedative anti-histamines can make the person drowsy and may even put him to sleep, which is often a good thing. But adults who take them must **not** drink alcohol, operate machinery or computers, or drive (in practice, travel sickness is very rare in drivers, since their minds are occupied).

The anti-spasm drugs are usually quicker acting. They may cause blurred vision, a dry mouth, difficulty in passing urine, and sometimes drowsiness. They too should not be taken by someone who is going to drive. DO NOT GIVE TO ANYONE WHO HAS GLAUCOMA.

Over-the-counter preparations for travel sickness include:

Avomine Sedative anti-histamine (promethazine).

Dramamine Sedative anti-histamine (dimenhydrinate).

Joy-Rides Contain anti-spasm drug hyoscine.

Kwells Contain anti-spasm drug hyoscine.

Kwells Junior Contains the same drug as Kwells (*see* above) at half the dose.

Marzine RF Sedative anti–histamine (cinnarzine).

Sea-Legs Sedative antihistamine (meclozine).

Stugeron Sedative anti-histamine (cinnarzine).

WARTS/VERRUCAS

GENERAL ADVICE
Verrucas are simply a type of wart which develops on the sole of the foot. All types of wart, including verrucas, are caused by viruses. This book, does not deal with warts on the sex organs (which should

always be treated by a doctor), only with warts on the skin and verrucas.

WARTS ON THE SKIN Many warts on the skin simply get better of their own accord, usually by withering and dropping off. However, if a wart is troublesome, or you find it unsightly, you can safely try any of the wart remedies listed in this section. Many of them contain a 'burning' agent, so please follow the directions on the label and keep the product well away from delicate parts of the body, especially the eyes.

WARNING: If you are in any doubt that the lump *is* a wart, please consult your doctor before treating it. This is particularly important if you are over 40.

VERRUCAS Unlike ordinary skin warts, these do not tend to get better on their own, and they can also cause pain.

There is much to be said for getting a verruca removed by a podiatrist or chiropodist, or (if one is available in your area) at a special verruca clinic that gets rid of them by freezing, burning or scraping (curetting). Although these procedures are usually done under local anaesthetic, they can be upsetting for children.

However, it is certainly justifiable to try and get rid of them with one of the over-the-counter remedies listed below. Be warned that treatment is not always successful at the first attempt.

Verrucas are infectious, so if the sufferer wants to go swimming she should wear a special 'verruca sock' that prevents the virus from getting onto the floor, and so being passed to other people.

NOTE: With all the products listed below take special care to follow the instructions on the pack, which are often quite complicated.

Over-the-counter preparations for warts and verrucas include:

Callusolve Wart Treatment For warts. Contains chloroform, liquid paraffin and benzalkonium chloride bromine. Apply after rubbing wart with pumice stone.

Carnation Verruca Treatment For verrucas. Dressing containing salicylic acid to be left on the verruca for two days.

Compound W For warts and verrucas. Liquid containing salicylic acid. Apply daily to wart or verruca for four weeks. Inflammable. A stronger preparation (Compound V) is available especially for verrucas.

Cuplex Gel For warts. Contains salicylic acid, lactic acid and copper. Soak the wart in hot water, then apply the gel as per instructions.

Duofilm Liquid For warts and verrucas. Contains salicylic acid and lactic acid. Apply after rubbing wart or verruca with a pumice stone.

Glutarol Wart Paint For warts and verrucas. Contains glutaraldehyde, methylated spirit and bitrex. Apply after rubbing wart or verruca with a pumice stone.

Novaruca For warts and verrucas. Contains glutaraldehyde. Apply twice daily and cover with a dressing.

Salactac Gel For warts. Main active ingredient is salicylic acid. Apply daily and rub wart once a week with special board provided.

Salactol Wart Paint For verrucas as well as warts. Contains salicylic acid, lactic acid and collodion. Follow directions carefully.

Veracur Gel For warts as well as verrucas.
Contains formaldehyde. Appy twice a day and cover
with a plaster.

Wartex Ointment For hard, rough warts. Contains
salicylic acid. Apply daily for several days, then
check with doctor.

WORMS

GENERAL ADVICE
Worms are common in children (and in adults in
many parts of the world), and are nothing to be
ashamed of. However, if somebody catches worms
there is usually some reason for it. So ask your
doctor if there is some way in which you can alter
your family's lifestyle or hygiene practices, in order
to prevent infection occurring again.

My feeling about worms it is always best to consult
a doctor, rather than treating the condition yourself.
However, there are some regions of the globe where
this is not practicable and where you may have to
go ahead and use self-treatment. This is particularly
justifiable if you are able to diagnose the *type* of
worm through previous experience.

Unfortunately, there are many different species of
worms which affect humans, and the type which
attacks your family will depend on the area of the
world in which you live. If it is not possible to get to
a doctor, a pharmacist may be able to help you with
diagnosis, and provide appropriate medication.

Over-the-counter preparations for worms include:

Alcopar Suitable for hookworm infestation. Sachets
containing bephenium. The effects of hookworm can
be so disastrous that you must make every effort to
obtain a doctor's advice.

Antepar Elixir For pinworms (threadworms) and roundworms. Pineapple-flavoured elixir containing piperazine, which may interfere with other drugs, and can cause incoordination ('worm wobble') and other side-effects. Do not use if you have epilepsy or kidney trouble.

Antepar Tablets Tablets containing the same ingredient as Antepar Elixir *(see* above*)*.

Ectodyne For pinworms (threadworms) and roundworms. Contains piperazine *(see* warnings under ***Antepar Elixir,*** above*)*.

Ovex For pinworms (threadworms). Chewable tablets containing mebendazole, which can cause tummy-ache and diarrhoea.

Pripsen Suitable for treating roundworms and pinworms (thread-worms). Powder containing senna and piperazine *(see* warnings under ***Antepar Elixir,*** above*)*.